MY REAL-WORLD GUIDE FOR EOSINOPHILIC ESOPHAGITIS.

MY REAL-WORLD GUIDE FOR EOSINOPHILIC ESOPHAGITIS

A guide to helping children, parents, and anyone else navigate through the thoughts and feelings associated with Eosinophilic Esophagitis.

DANIELLE TRAVIS

Copyright © 2015 Danielle Travis
All rights reserved.

ISBN: 1506028373
ISBN 13: 9781506028378

A NOTE:

Before I begin, I want to tell everyone about the cover. You may be wondering what the EoE is made out of. Well, my brother (Matthew), carved that out of a block of wood and then painted it purple (my favorite color). I have the best brother ever.

Also, I would like to thank a lot of people (cause when else will I get the cool opportunity to do this). Of course, my parents and brother for supporting me, emotionally, financially, and physically. You have truly always been my number one fans. You have done more for me than I will ever be able to express on paper -thank you.

James: I'm so happy to have you in my life. Thank you for loving and supporting me through all of the ups and downs.

Rachel: You've been my BFF since 9th grade. Thank you for being the sister I never had.

To Alexi and Allie: Thank you for taking the time to flip through each page and give me amazing critique. I couldn't have finished this book without your thoroughness and precision to detail.

I'd like to say thank you to all of my other friends and family. Whether you know it or not, you've all made an impression on my life that I'll always carry with me.

I'd also like to thank Jesus. He listens to me and always has my back.

And finally, to all of the people who made fun of my formula, to the people who whispered behind my back, and to the people who discouraged me---thank you for the motivation.

WARNING:

This book is not a substitute for a doctor. I am a college student, not a doctor. This book is not designed to make medical decisions, but is a "feelings" book. I will try to help you understand the emotions that go on behind the scenes and how your child may feel.

I wish I could have talked to someone around my age that had been through this to know what it was going to be like. To help other people who are either going through this, or who are struggling with the decision to go through with it or not.

Also: For Eosinophilic Esophagitis, there are many options for attempting to handle this disease. While I discuss many options throughout the book, I do not go into detail about steroid treatment. I never had steroid treatment, and therefore don't have any experiences to talk about it.

TABLE OF CONTENTS

Introduction · xi
My Family and My Background · xiii
My Early Childhood Memories · xv
Part 1 When I could eat some food, however limited it may be · · 1
May I Take Your Order? · 3
Let's see if You Have What it Takes · 5
It's Okay to Cry · 8
Plain and Simple Hatred · 9
Angels in Scrubs · 11
America Doesn't Even Know What A Vegetable Is. · · · · · · · · · · 12
The One Who Stood Out · 14
Organize, It's Crucial · 15
Cheater Cheater Pumpkin Eater
(Unless You're Allergic to Pumpkin) · 16
"I Don't Like This or That…or Anything for That Matter." · · · · 19
Here We Go Again · 20
Thanksgiving in January · 22
The Good, the Bad, and the Ugly · 23
Part 2 The no-food liquid elemental diet. · · · · · · · · · · · · · · · 25
Bangin' Like Britney · 27
Formula Importance · 29
A Monster in Disguise · 32
Be Your Own Role Model · 33
One Day Down · 34

A Little Sugar Goes a Long Way · 36
The Parentals · 37
The Siblings · 38
Smells always have the Same Effect · · · · · · · · · · · · · · · · · · · 39
The Strongest Sick One · 41
Happy Mother's Day · 43
Ahh, Fresh Air · 45
Loud and Proud · 48
Just a Little Bitter · 50
Thanksgiving in May · 52
Become A Busy Bee · 53
Just Count Backwards from 100 · 55
Journey (not the song, silly) · 58
To Go Elemental or Not? That is the Question. · · · · · · · · · 59
Part 3 (The part adding food back on one at a time) · · · · · · **61**
Introduction · 63
This or That, Doc? · 64
Definition of Weakness · 66
The Devil is Everywhere · 68
Conclusion · 71
Part 4 (Another Diagnosis) · **73**
Wait…What? · 75
So, what is it? · 76
Am I breaking? · 77
So now what? · 80
Part 5 (The technical part) · **81**
Deathly Hallows of Insurance · 83
How to Handle the Holidays (or any special event.) · · · · · · · 85
Stereotypes: Therapy · 86
The Sweet Seven · 88
Remember Me! · 90
A Brief Story · 92
References · 95
The…No, I Don't Want it to be the End · · · · · · · · · · · · · · · 97

INTRODUCTION

Hello to all reading this book. You may be reading this because like me, you're someone who has food allergies, and you want to know more about someone you might be able to relate to. Maybe you're a concerned parent, wondering what truly goes through the mind of your suffering 15 year old with severe food allergies. Or maybe you're just curious and want to know more about my experiences.

For whatever reason you're reading this book, I can assure you that it's the honest truth. This book has been four years in the making. I started writing when I was 16 years old, and I wrote a little bit here and a little bit there. I am now 20 years old, and I'm finally finished! This book will give you an inside look at what my experiences have been living with food allergies, what I've found to get through the rough spots, and how I've come to live at peace with my diagnosis and symptoms in the long run. In this book I will not tell you that I understand how you feel, tell you that you have it better than a lot of other people, or tell you to make lemonade out of lemons. I will however tell you how I've found living with food allergies sucks, how easy it is to get depressed without your favorite foods, and how I have managed to cope. It is my hope that reading this will prepare you for what you might encounter; if you have just been diagnosed with food allergies or EoE, or perhaps it will help you connect better with your son or daughter who is going through this living hell in everyday life, or maybe this will simply help you learn about life from another person's perspective. Whatever your reason is for reading this, I hope that I can help through my stories. This book is designed to educate you in the basic knowledge of food allergies and food-related diseases.

There are five parts to my book: the first four parts of more of an inside look into my thoughts and feelings. If you're trying to understand how your child might be feeling, or if you're looking to relate to someone else, then this is for you. Part one includes edited stories I wrote when I was on an elimination diet and could eat a few select foods. Part two are stories I wrote when I was on an elemental diet, and could not eat any food at all, but was on a liquid diet instead. Part three are stories I wrote when I was in the process of adding foods back into my diet one at a time from the elemental diet. Part four are stories and thoughts from when I was diagnosed with something called Ehlers-Danlos Syndrome. Finally, part five is the technical part where I give some quick last minute tips. There's a page to check out some really helpful websites and a really cool story.

For each part, there aren't any chapters. Instead, each new "piece" is a diary entry on a specific topic. It's about how I was feeling at the time and what I was thinking. Underneath the diary entry, you'll see: "Tips and Tricks" and "Word to the Wise." The "Tips and Tricks" is a piece of advice for a child (or someone who is has Eosinophilic Esophagitis) to take away from the diary entry. The "Word to the Wise" is a piece of advice for the parents (or someone who is helping someone along the process) on the specific topic.

Throughout the book, I also include a few pictures from my life. Just to give you a little more of an inside look and to give you some visual representation!

I hope you use this as a tool to help you navigate through the sticky situations that you may encounter. I know I wish I had had something to guide me through the tough decisions. I hope this helps!

MY FAMILY AND MY BACKGROUND

So, some of you may be asking what I was like in my past. Did I just randomly wake up allergic one-day and not able to eat chicken? The answer to your question is no. I've had food allergies my entire life. If you're a parent reading this book, and you have a small child with food allergies, then you may want to pay attention to some of this because these anecdotes could be signs of problems you might encounter in the future.

Before I get into my story, it's important that you know that I have a history of food problems within my family. My great uncle had reflux, then Barrett's esophagus, and then contracted throat cancer. He passed

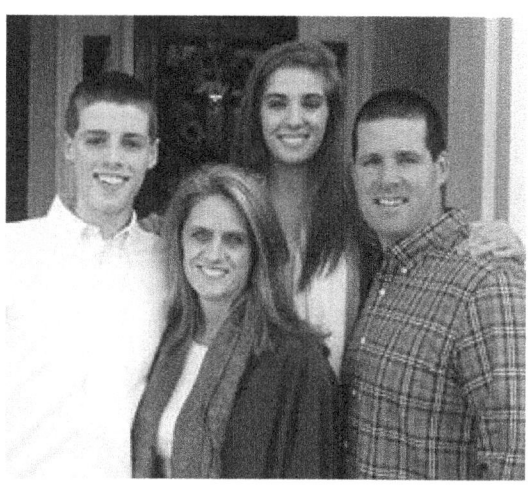

Above is a picture of the people behind all of the magic. My mom, the one who cooked all of my weird foods and constantly sat in on appointments with me. My dad, who was always my pillar of strength and solid rock foundation. And, my brother, who always knew how to put a smile on my face and is one of the most thoughtful people that I know.

away shortly after he was diagnosed, as the cancer took over. My dad has had several scopes done, and he has strictures and harsh reflux. My grandfather, before having surgery, had colon cancer. Look at your family history to see if you're at an increased risk to have gastrointestinal problems in the future. Your chances are going to become a lot higher if you come from a line of people with food problems.

My food problems started the day I was born. I couldn't keep milk down, and I would throw everything up. My mom nicknamed me "The Vomit Machine" because that's exactly what I would do. Anything that went down was guaranteed to come right back up. The doctors diagnosed me with severe acid reflux and finally, after months of switching formulas, we found one that my body could tolerate, and relief was in sight.

So that whole part above is obviously not from my recollection; it's stories from my mom. But this part- these are all my accounts from the earliest age I can remember.

MY EARLY CHILDHOOD MEMORIES

Skip ahead a few years and I'm three years old. My mom has just bought me a chicken sandwich for lunch; I took one bite of it and told her I didn't want to eat it anymore. I couldn't explain the feeling, but I knew it hurt and I didn't want to finish the sandwich. My mom thought I was just being a typical picky three year old, and told me to eat my lunch. Well, a couple of minutes later, my lunch was all over the floor. Parents, pay attention to this. If your child is telling you they don't want to eat something, please don't automatically assume it's because they're being picky. Perhaps if your child simply cannot explain why they don't want to eat a food, there may be something else going on.

When I was about seven or eight years old. My mom had made me some turkey rolls and a chocolate chip cookie. Once again, I told my mom that I didn't want to eat the turkey rolls, but I did want the cookie. She said that if I wanted the cookie, then I had to eat the turkey. So, being a kid, I forced down the turkey just to get the cookie. With each bite of turkey, my pain got worse and worse. My throat was itchy, my face was flushed, and it hurt to swallow. But I was a kid, and I didn't know that that pain was abnormal. I thought all people experienced that sort of discomfort when eating turkey. And besides, I wanted that cookie.

It wasn't until I was about 9 years old that I was finally able to explain to my mom that when I ate certain foods I got an "itchy throat," I told her I just wanted to reach my hand down into my throat and scratch it because it was really itchy. (Parents, listen to little signs like this, because they're usually an indicator that something bigger is going on).

My mom took me to an allergist who gave me a whole list of possible allergens. She said that all this would probably pass and I would be able to eat things like chicken again when I was 15 or 16. I am 16 now, turning 17 in two months and chicken is still one of my worst foods.

As I got older, I found out through trial and error which foods I had to avoid. The list included: chicken, turkey, lettuce, tomato, nuts, and fresh fruit. I know it's a very odd assortment, but it's what worked for me.

Pretty soon, I was having more and more "itchy throats". Sometimes they got pretty serious, and I would have to go to the ER. In addition, I was having more and more reactions to foods I used to be fine with; pizza, brownies and sandwiches were all starting to bother me. Also, I started becoming scared to eat food, because my throat was closing whenever I tried a new or random food. I didn't know what foods were "safe". Therefore, I would rather not eat or just eat rice cereal. After multiple doctors, my parents then took me to a gastroenterologist at age 14. He listened to my stories, and he thought I had a disease called, "Eosinophilic Esophagitis" (EoE). He explained to me how new the disease was, and how it was diagnosed.

A couple of months later, I got my first endoscopy. When the results came back, my throat was covered with eosinophils. Eosinophils are the white blood cells found in your esophagus (throat) that cause all the inflammation and problems. The doctors said I had Eosinophilic Esophagitis. The doctor told us the treatment options, telling us all about the elimination diet, the elemental diet, and the steroids (I'll explain all the options in more depth later on). He told us that scopes were going to have to happen every three months. My parents couldn't bear to hear that I would have to have an endoscope every three months. But, we went ahead with a non-traditional elimination diet. Traditionally, elimination diets are where the top eight food allergens are taken out of the diet. That includes shellfish, peanuts, tree-nuts, wheat, milk, eggs, fish, and soy. I, on the other hand, did an elimination diet based on everything that came back positive from my food allergy testing. Some of these foods were rice, corn, wheat, and oats. This eliminated a big majority of foods and my daily diet consisted of foods like beef, ham, green beans, potatoes, and some types of vanilla ice cream. Now, let me say this: Just because a food comes back positive on the allergy testing, **does not mean you are allergic to it**. It is well known that allergy testing is not 100% accurate. I only wish my doctor would have told me this before I took off all of these foods.

During the summer before my 9th grade year, I went on this elimination diet. Right before school came back in, I got my second scope. When the results came back, almost all of the eosinophils were gone. I was so overjoyed and overwhelmed. Over the course of the summer, I had only one allergic reaction! This was amazing considering that a few months before, I had had an allergic reaction about once a week. I was so relieved that I pretty much went back to my regular diet. I was perfectly okay with this at the time because I couldn't stand the thought of not having my favorite foods any longer. This would prove to be a big mistake later down the road, and I would regret this decision and come to find out that eating my favorite foods just led to more frustration and complications.

For the next two years, I went back to my regular diet. I would eat anything I wanted with the exception of things I hadn't eaten since I was three, like chicken, lettuce, and tomato. My allergies came back too. I started having to go home more often from school because the pain was unbearable. I had to visit the nurse every other day at lunch, and had to take more and more Benadryl. My parents and I were both getting tired of this; allergic reactions aren't fun. They are scary and exhausting. We went to appointments after appointments, trying to figure my body out. We went to homeopathic doctors, allergists; you name it, and we probably went there.

We had all reached our breaking points when I had to be taken to the hospital one afternoon. I had eaten a roast beef sandwich for lunch. I then went to the gym, and on my way back from the gym, my throat started to close; I couldn't breathe. I drove home safely and got my brother to call my dad. My dad came home and then rushed me to the E.R.

After that hospital trip, my parents and I both knew something had to be done. My mom and dad looked around a little bit, checking out different specialty doctors and hospitals. The doctors at my local hospital recommended Cincinnati Children's Hospital. Cincinnati Children's hospital is one that specializes in Eosinophilic disorders. I asked my dad if we could call and check it out and we began researching the hospital and how it worked. Basically, new patients come in for a week evaluation, and then at the end of the week the whole family and a team of doctors sit down and figure out a plan of action. After my dad told me this, I felt so happy, so relieved. I was happy that we finally had a plan. A plan that I could follow.

After months of waiting it was finally our time to go to Cincinnati. Let me just say this, Cincinnati Children's Hospital is amazing. I give my total recommendation to it. The doctors are highly qualified, the nurses are extremely helpful, and the whole experience was a positive one. My scope went wonderfully; the anesthesiologists are wonderful. Having about a few endoscopes under my belt, I knew a good team of doctors, and this team of doctors has been the best by far. At the end of the week, we met with my main doctor and discussed the game plan. He basically gave ME three options. I capitalize me because, for once, the doctors there asked what I wanted. They listened to *me*, and talked to *me*. They were so attentive and wanted to include me in the decisions. The three options were: an elimination diet of the top eight food allergies in children, an elemental diet, or steroids. In the end we chose the eight-food elimination diet, with a plan to see the hospital again in three months to get my second scope.

I left Cincinnati feeling refreshed and hopeful.

About six weeks into my elimination diet, weird things started to happen. I wasn't really having allergic reactions, but I was having food stuck in my throat, all the time. My mom kept telling me to take slower bites, but it didn't matter how many times I chewed before I swallowed, the food was sticking in my throat. My parents talked to the doctors in Cincinnati, and after careful thought, we decided to go on the elemental diet. I keep on using the pronoun "we" because it was a "we" kind of decision. My parents don't just make all the decisions for me, and I didn't just decide everything and they go along with it. One of the most important things is talking about it with your family, discussing every option and every decision. I know that it's not always fun talking, and you guys will probably disagree on a lot of stuff, but that's okay. I remember crying after discussing things with my parents, not because I was mad at them, but because I was just mad at my situation.

My point in telling you some of my background information is to just give you an insight as to what road your child may be heading down and what signs you may want to pay attention to.

PART 1
(WHEN I COULD EAT SOME FOOD, HOWEVER LIMITED IT MAY BE)

MAY I TAKE YOUR ORDER?

One of the most hindering and inconvenient things about food problems is the lack of food on the go. Whether it was track and field, youth group, babysitting, frisbee with friends, or running for president (just kidding), I'm always on the go! So where does lunch fit into this? 90% of the population would grab a chicken sandwich, a cheeseburger, or maybe a salad. Given my condition, that simply doesn't work for me, but it's pretty difficult to bring a whole cooler and pack some rice pasta, and then find a public microwave. So what do I do? Well, I make friends with the people at Wendy's, Hardee's, Subway, and Arby's. When I was younger, I found one of my better qualities was making friends. I'm so glad I do, because it's really paying off now. Now, it's easy to order a quick hamburger patty and fries not touched with the other food (I could eat the plain beef patty but not the bread or any condiments that came along with it). In the beginning, it was frustrating. They would give me weird looks and get my order wrong. But, as I started to come back, the workers started to recognize me, and would greet me with a smile. My favorite place so far has been Hardee's, where I've found they have the biggest patty for the lowest price.

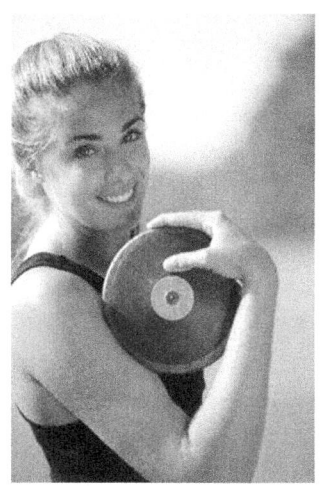

I loved being on the go, and I loved discus!

A Tip and a Trick: When placing a special order at a new restaurant for the first time, be patient. The cashier or waitress may get it wrong the first or second time, but as you go back, your order will be remembered and instead of weird looks, they'll start to give you a friendly smile.

Word to the Wise: Parents- encourage your child to eat with the family whenever possible. Eating at a restaurant will not only bring a smile to your child's face, but it can be a new way to get an old food, which is always fun. Just make sure that their food is cooked separately and with different utensils.

LETS SEE IF YOU HAVE WHAT IT TAKES

When I was on the eight-food elimination diet, I was pretty restricted in what I ate. This diet took out all wheat, milk, shellfish, peanuts, tree nuts, fish, soy, and egg, plus the stuff that I've never been able to eat like lettuce, tomato, chicken, turkey, and fresh fruit, and you have quite a list. Taking away all of these foods required a lot of flexibility. For example, when my mom would make me a cake, she would use rice flour (wheat substitute), rice milk (milk substitute), sunflower oil (butter substitute), and egg substitute (made from tapioca flour). Anyways, when I had to have a lot of substitutes, foods didn't always come out of the oven the way they were supposed to. Breads and cakes didn't rise; soups didn't have the same color, etc. Being allergic to so many things, I didn't mind the strange colors, the weird looks, or the odd smells. As long as it tasted somewhat decent and I was allowed to have it, I would eat it. Around the time I was in the tenth grade, I was sitting at the lunch table and everyone saw my interesting food. They would joke about the food I ate, calling it baby food, saying it was smelly, make gagging sounds. Even though I knew they were kidding, there's always a little truth behind every joke. They knew I couldn't really help eating what I had to eat, but that didn't seem to slow down their jokes.

I'm the type of person who can laugh at myself, and for a while I went along with their snide comments and questionable jokes. I laughed when people asked why I had dog food for lunch and played along when someone would casually move away from me because they didn't want to be near my food. But pretty soon I started to get tired of it. I knew that if I tried to explain why my food looked different from everybody else's, they would get confused and just wouldn't understand. I knew that to shut some people up, I had to show them how difficult my situation actually was. So I got to thinking. I thought, and I thought, and I thought. Finally, I came up with the perfect idea. People had no idea the "shoes" I was in, so, why not put them in my shoes? I also knew how much people like a challenge, so that's exactly what I was going to give them.

The next day, I created a Facebook event called, "Eat like Danielle for a Week". Under the description, I put that this was just to support people with food allergies, and how I thought it would be interesting. I then listed my food allergies with examples of what foods contained wheat, what some of my favorite foods were, and what labels were tricky to read. I set the event for a week, seeing how many people were going to be up for the challenge.

Anyways, I set the date and then watched while, slowly but surely, more and more people joined the event. The day before the event started, around 20 of my peers had signed up to accept the challenge. Going through the week, people came up to me and told me how hard the challenge was for them. They told me how they were going to eat that brownie last night, but then thought of me and put it down. They said that they thought I was really cool for what I had to go through. In addition to admiration, people also came up to me and complained to me. They told me how hungry they were. At the lunch table, they told me how badly they wanted some pizza. *Well now you know how I feel every single day*, I would say to myself.

By the end of the week, I believe only a few of the 20 managed to complete the challenge. You would think that I'd be disappointed that only a few actually stuck through it, but I was actually very pleased with the end results. Just because some people didn't finish it, or even start it, a lot of people did gain a whole new respect for me. They got a glimpse of understanding. After that, the comments about my food went down to a bare minimum. So, I got their respect without having to seem like a person who "couldn't take a joke".

A Tip and a Trick: If people are making jokes about your food or teasing you about it, don't let it slide. I did for too long, and it didn't benefit me at all. Use my idea, or find your own way give people a glimpse into your life. If you use my idea about getting people to eat like you, I suggest that you set it for a day, or maybe just a few days. An entire week was a little too much for most people.

Word to the Wise: I know it's hard to hear about your child being teased at lunch. Try to listen and just support your child and encourage them to take a stand.

IT'S OKAY TO CRY

No matter how strong you are, sometimes you have to cry. Now, I know that everyone deals with stress in his or her own way, but sometimes, you just have to cry. I cried because I felt out of control and I didn't know what was going to happen next. I remember going up to my room, closing my door quietly, crying, wiping my tears on the wall, and then going back downstairs, feeling fresh and rejuvenated. I know sometimes my parents wouldn't understand why I was crying. They would get frustrated and tell me not to worry; sometimes they would blame my tears on exhaustion. Granted, sometimes I was tired, but other times, I just needed to cry. Crying is healthy. Crying is good. It shows that your heart is beating, hurting, healing, and loving. Sometimes I feel like I want to curl up in a ball and forget about this world. I want to forget about this world that's full of yummy smells and exotic foods. Then I remember how many people love and adore me. And that makes me crawl out of my hole. I believe crying is one of the best ways to relieve stress. Sometimes it just feels like allergies and diseases are too much to handle.

A Tip and a Trick: Just let it out. I know how hard it is for you and I know the stress you're dealing with. Take a deep breath and know that you'll get through this.

Word to the Wise: Tell your children that they can cry if they want to. Don't make them feel ashamed or like they have to hide it. And don't be afraid to cry in front of your child. Let them know that when they're in pain, you're in pain. But also remember, while it feels like your world is crumbling, know that it'll get better. This disease is very livable once you get it under control.

PLAIN AND SIMPLE HATRED

I hate Eosinophilic Esophagitis. I hate it so much. It brings me pain, it brings my family pain, it brings hospital bills, it brings fights, and it brings worry. Because I am on the elimination diet, I'm getting food stuck in my throat all of the time. It's pretty painful, and I can't do anything about it except wait for it to pass. The pain I feel is like if you're trying to swallow a golf ball, and yet you can't; it just kind of sits there in your throat until my saliva slides it down.

This is where I am in the process; my dad is going to talk to my doctor to see what we should do next.

I start to cry, wondering why God chose me to bear this burden. I mean, I don't blame God. In fact, I don't blame anyone for this. I feel like my parents sometimes feel responsible for me having EoE. They feel like if they had done something differently when I was young, that this could have somehow been prevented. I don't think so, I think it's how the cards of life played out, and I don't blame anybody. My parents seem so mad, so frustrated. They wanted this elimination diet to work, and now my body is screwing it up. I feel like I should say I'm sorry. Please excuse my body for being difficult; I'll try to get a healthier one next time. It seems like I bring such a burden to my parents. Neither mom nor dad wants to do the elemental diet, but what choice do we have left?

This elimination diet is supposed to work. I'm supposed to eliminate the eight main food groups, and everything is supposed to get better. But no, my body had to cause a riot. This is another one of the downers of this disease, or any disease for that matter. Not only does this bring me physical pain, but also it really does put so much tension on my family. True, some nights are better than others, but I just wish there weren't any bad nights.

I think I get so angry because it seems like I've come to a dead end. I was so mad, and then Cincinnati came, and it opened up a new path. But still, after Cincinnati, it seems like I'm rounding the corner, about to come to that familiar dead end.

I do have some faith in the elemental diet. I mean, that has to work. That is the last resort. The best way to describe it is bittersweet. It's something that I know will work, (as in clearing the eosinophils) but it's bitter because of how difficult it is to keep such a strict diet.

Thanks for taking the time to read this chapter. This chapter helped me by making me turn my anger into words. It made me feel better.

A Tip and a Trick: I know you get angry sometimes. Go do something about it. See what I just did above? I wrote. I expressed my anger and got it out of my system. Find a way to express yours.

Word to the Wise: I know you get just as angered with the failure of a diet. I know you get angry when you see that your child is frustrated. But don't give up. There's always something else to try. Have faith.

ANGELS IN SCRUBS

It's critical to find your silver linings. A big silver lining for me has been Smarty's (the candy). I was thinking the other day when I was filling out a scholarship application about what I want to study in college. I'm pretty sure that I want to be a pediatric nurse. Some people are surprised that I'm so specific and so adamant about what I want to do, but I think it's the career for me. Because I've had allergic reactions and attacks, I've made one or two trips to the emergency room. That's always been a rough time in my life, each night is very scary, but I will always remember will be the nurses that helped me. You would think that I'd remember the doctors more, the people that actually gave me the medicine to stop my throat from closing, but no, the nurses are the ones that helped calm me down, who listened to me, and who even understood some of my pain. I believe that nurses are the silver linings of a hospital.

When I go to college, I want to study nursing. I want to be a nurse so I can have the opportunity to show the kindness and love that so many nurses have shown me. This is my permanent way of saying thank you to all of the nurses out there who have made my hospital trips a little less scary and a little more bearable.

A Tip and a Trick: Have patience when you run into a bad nurse. You know, the one who pricks you five times before they finally stick the needle into your arm. And when you run into that really good, sweet, kind nurse, be sure to tell her you truly appreciate her.

Word to the Wise: Be sure to let your child's voice be heard. When he or she is old enough, let them talk to the nurses themselves. It will not only give him or her confidence, but will make them feel a sense of control. I always enjoyed talking to my nurses, instead of being talked about.

AMERICA DOESN'T EVEN KNOW WHAT A VEGETABLE IS

America is obsessed with food. I'll say it loud and proud. **America is obsessed with food.** I don't care how fat, skinny, healthy, or unhealthy you are, chances are, you're obsessed with food too. I know I still am, even though I can only be obsessed with a small list of foods. If we don't get the foods we crave, we can become frustrated. If we don't like a taste, no matter how beneficial it is to our body, we won't eat it.

Just the other day, I walked by a teacher in my school that was throwing an absolute hissy fit because she did not get the exact lunch she ordered. Boo hoo. People have forgotten that food is not here to please us. Food is not here to make us happy. Food should not determine our mood, nor should food be the center focal point of our social interactions. Think about it: When you want to see an old friend, what do you say? "Want to meet up for lunch?" My personal belief is that food has one main purpose; food is here to give us the nutrients we need to live. Our body is like a machine. We have to feed the machine in order for it to keep running. When you add gunk to the machine, it moves slower and has to have more repairs. When you add high quality stuff to the machine, it runs smoother and lasts longer. To me: oatmeal pies, cheeseburgers, ice cream, and pancakes are the cheap, gunk stuff. Vegetables, lean meats, fruits, and whole grains are the high quality, good stuff that will keep your body going for a pretty long time. Now, for anyone who has to go on the elemental diet (the liquid one that I will get into in part 2), think of the formula as straight powerhouse super formula. You may hate the taste but it's exactly what your body needs. I remember that I would wake up in the morning and crave some peach oatmeal.

Oooh yes, I said to myself as I walked downstairs. I'm going to get me some peach oatmeal. As I was opening the cabinet, I could already taste the peaches on my tongue. I could feel the slick oatmeal sliding down, warming my stomach. And then, what do you know, we're out of oatmeal. What do I do? I go yell at my mom asking why she didn't buy more oatmeal when she was at the grocery store. I failed to realize that toast would give me the same number of calories and would fill my body in the same way. I, like many Americans, was blinded by the taste. And that is my point of how completely obsessive we can get over food.

I wish we, as a country, could get over our obsession with food. I wish we would see it for what it truly is. I believe that we would be a happier, healthier society if we focused more on our relationships and less on what was in the refrigerator.

A Tip and a Trick: Like I mentioned above, I used to get upset with my mom when I ran out of my favorite food. Give her a break once in a while. She's trying her best and it's not all about food.

Word to the Wise: If you're trying to raise your kids with a good perspective, teach them that life is not about eating. I truly do believe that America is too focused on eating, and it's caused us a lot of problems.

THE ONE WHO STOOD OUT

I'm nearing the end of my junior year and I'm starting to fill out applications for college scholarships. They ask all the usual questions about my personal goals and accomplishments: what I want to be when I get older, how I make a difference in my community, etc. In order to stand out as an applicant, I knew I would have to make my essays jump off the page. Now, what better way to stand out than to talk about my allergies? It's something very unique, something that is a personal accomplishment each day, and it gives me a lot of different perspectives. When I write or talk about my food allergies, I'm showing my uniqueness and telling the world how I embrace it.

Recently, I applied for a free trip to Washington, D.C. to represent my state at a youth conference. I mentioned my disease briefly on my application, and when I got called in for an interview, the judges asked me about it. They first asked me what Eosinophilic Esophagitis was, then they asked me about my outlook on life because of it and how I overcame the disabilities it presented me. All of these questions, and the answers to my questions, not only told them about my disease, but it told them about how I tried to live my life; it told them about my personal character.

A Tip and a Trick: When writing an essay for any college or scholarship, make them stand out; make the admissions office remember you. Use your disadvantages to your advantage and make them look twice at your application.

Word to the Wise: When your child is feeling down about what he or she has to live through, emphasis how unique and special it makes them. While it's not the ideal way to stand out, it still makes them very unique. Help them realize that they have been given something that can help others. That's exactly what I realized when I started writing this. I have something that makes me stand out, so let me use my voice and make something out of it.

ORGANIZE, ITS CRUCIAL

Parents, this section is really for you. One very important, critical key in whatever stage you're going through is *organization*. I cannot tell you how important this is. Keep every paper the doctors hand you, every bill that's mailed to you, write down all the phone calls you have, and keep all the notes you write. I'm so thankful that my mom is naturally an organizer. She started when I was just a baby. She got a big blue folder and just started keeping everything. This turned out to be really important because numerous times the hospital would mess up the billing information and charge us with stuff that clearly wasn't ours. Hospitals and doctors have a bunch of different numbers and sometimes they can get pretty confusing. My mom kept a sheet with all the direct lines to my specific doctors. Those really came in handy. If you have everything together, things will seem a little more in your control and you'll feel a little better. This wasn't a really long section, but it is a very important section.

A Tip and a Trick: I know when I was younger; I used to poke fun at my mom for hauling that big blue folder around to every appointment. But now, looking back on it, I am eternally thankful for her. Remember to thank your parents for everything they do; it's not easy to be the parent of someone with Eosinophilic Esophagitis.

Word to the Wise: I don't mean to repeat myself, but I really feel strongly about this. Keep all of your documents including: medicine records, sensitivities to foods, previous appointments, questions, etc.

CHEATER CHEATER PUMPKIN EATER (UNLESS YOU'RE ALLERGIC TO PUMPKINS)

I walk into our local Kroger, 30 minutes before school starts, and head straight to the "Nature's Market" section. I'm amazingly familiar with this section, knowing which side the soy milk is on and which brand of rice puffs are the best. I quickly grab a box of raisins and vitamin water and make my way to the cash register. I would usually eat some dry rice cereal before school, but it was just one of those mornings.

As I make my way to the register, I pass by a stand of granola bars. A simple box of chocolate chip granola bars, store brand. A 1.99 a box, nothing amazing, nothing spectacular. But to me and to anyone who can't have them, it's a 1.99 box of gold. I swallow as I remember the taste of a chocolate chip granola bar I had 9 months ago. Chewy, salty at first, and then sweet as your tongue went over the chocolate chips. I back up a few steps and just look at them. I know I can't have them. One of two things would happen: I would either have an allergic reaction, my throat would start to close, and I would be in bed all day. Or, nothing physical could happen, and I would just ruin the trial. What I mean by trial is that when I would get a scope in three months, I may get false results back if I eat food that I'm not supposed to have. I stand there, and next thing you know, that box of granola bars is in my hand. "This is a bad idea" I say to myself as I bit my lip and ponder over whether or not to take the chance.

Now, if you're the type of person reading this book, and you don't have food issues, then you're probably thinking I'm insane right now. Who would possibly risk their life for a stupid little granola bar? Who would take the chance? Well, for someone who eats rice and corn all day, a granola bar is heaven. A granola bar, that taste, makes you feel better inside. It fills that hole. Well, I grabbed that box and practically ran to the register. I kept looking over my shoulder, feeling guilty, knowing I was committing one of the highest sins. I pay for it in cash, not wanting this abhorrence to show up permanently on my debit card statement. I tell the clerk that I don't need a bag, thinking in my head that I'll probably throw the rest of the box away; I just want that one granola bar. As I get into my car, I hesitate once more. I know this is a bad idea. But today, rash decisions overtake my common sense and I open the wrapper and stuff the bar into my mouth. As I'm chewing, I'm thinking about what I have just done. I have officially screwed up my trial. I swallow in frustration, regretting it all. The glorious taste isn't worth the suffering, the pain, or the confusion. Once again, my mind played tricks on me. Or, better yet, my taste buds played tricks on me. Sighing, I start my car and pull into the street, ready to start my school day. To sum everything else up: I didn't get a reaction, and am so thankful I didn't. I was so ashamed, so embarrassed by my weakness. In fact, I didn't tell anyone. I just wanted to forget my failure and move on. The rest of the day, I felt dirty. I vowed that I would never cheat again. It wasn't worth it. But, as I now know writing this, that that wouldn't be my last time to cheat, nor would it be my last time feeling like a failure.

The moral of this story is not to tell you not to cheat. I realize that if you go on an elimination diet, if you have bad allergies, you will be tempted to cheat. And unless you have the will power of a robot, then I also realize that you probably will cheat. While I do not want anyone to cheat on his or her diet, I realize that it's a possibility. I had to figure it out on my own that I'm not perfect, and that I will mess up. After I would cheat, I would feel weak, and stupid, and hopeless.

A Tip and a Trick: After you cheat, recognize that it's truly not worth it. Believe me, I know the temptation. I go through it every day. And remember that when you're hunched over, shoveling that granola bar in, or maybe picking a piece of brownie off of the last tray, remember that you're not alone. Remember that there are other people who are struggling right along with you. Also, if you do slip up, talk to your parents about it. I know, it may sound impossible. Why would you voluntarily tell your parents every time you do something illegal? I know it sounds hard, but you should do it. I know I didn't, but I think if I had, it would have helped me cope a lot. I was so embarrassed about my failure that I would just keep it bottled up inside, only getting madder at myself. Just because you give in to temptation, doesn't mean you're weak and a failure. It just means that you're learning from your mistakes.

Word to the Wise: If you catch your child cheating, or if they come to you and tell you that they ate something that they weren't supposed to, take a deep breath. Yes, it sucks. They've either messed up a scope date or hurt their bodies or both. It's not only time-consuming but it's money consuming. It benefits no one and only frustrates you more. I get it. But please, realize how difficult of a time your child is having. In a perfect world, sneaking food wouldn't even be a thing. And yet, in the world of EoE, it seems criminal to take a bite of chocolate. When (not if) your child sneaks food, talk to them. Explain how it hurts not only their bodies, but also the process of healing them. Ask them why they wanted to sneak food; were the hungry? Upset? Lonely? If they cheat when they're hungry, try leaving their "safe" food in an easy to reach spot. If they're upset, leave out paper and pencil so they can write down their feelings, and have them throw it in a basket and hopefully that can replace cheating. Figure out the emotions behind the cheating, so you can try to prevent the cheating.

"I DON'T LIKE THIS OR THAT...OR ANYTHING FOR THAT MATTER"

One of my biggest pet peeves ever would probably be a picky eater. I cannot stand someone who chooses with their free will to not eat a food because they don't like the taste. This is especially an annoyance for me, since I'm extremely limited in the food I eat. I just don't understand why someone would voluntarily not eat a food. It just doesn't make sense to me. Now, I've never been a picky eater, so I don't know exactly what I'm talking about, but it seems pretty simple to me. Some of my friends are picky eaters. I watch them take one bite or just even one smell or look at something, and then they wouldn't eat it. I watch in madness as they smelled a food and then put it down, refusing to try it. Maybe they're so picky because they have the luxury of that freedom to be picky. They can pick and choose what foods fit their exact palate and still have plenty to choose from. Oh the jealousy.

A Tip and a Trick: I know how annoying it is when you have friends that are picky eaters, believe me I get it. Just breathe through it and tell them that they're lucky and shouldn't take advantage of that fact.

Word to the Wise: When your child has a friend over, try introducing them to some of your child's food. If you present it in a fun way, they may like it and learn to expand their palate.

HERE WE GO AGAIN

One of the most annoying and repetitive things about having food problems or food-related disease would be explaining it to other people. Not only is it difficult to explain to someone why you can't eat that while they casually chow down, but it's even harder to explain it in a timely manner so you don't lose their attention. They just don't understand at first. And then comes the repetition. Once you teach and tell them enough times, they slowly but surely start to understand. I am forced to tell people daily about my disease and explain myself. I say forced because I really don't want to, I just get tired of saying the same thing over and over again.

Sometimes when I tell people about this disease that I have, they ask me if I'm going to die. Well, I think to myself, of course. Everyone dies. You'll probably die before me because of your unhealthy eating habits. But obviously I never say this. Instead, I explain it to them this way: "Having this disease is just like having something like diabetes. When someone has diabetes, you can't tell. They don't stick out from a crowd and they can get their disease under control. Now, there will be some scary moments, like when your blood sugar gets too low and you pass out, but usually everything will be okay. That's just the way this disease works, you can't tell that I have it, and once I figure out what foods I can and cannot have, I'll live just as long as anyone else."

A Tip and a Trick: So, you may ask how's the best way to tell someone about your disease. I would say try to dumb it down a lot, not because the people are dumb, but because the subject matter is so complicated. Also, the more times you have to explain what you have, the quicker you'll get at it. I remember when I first had to tell people why I could have beef but not chicken; I would go into this 20-minute monologue and I could tell that in the first five minutes they had stopped listening. But now, through lots and lots of practice, I can sum up food allergies, Eosinophilic Esophagitis, and elemental diet in 45 seconds. It's definitely an accomplishment of mine. Here's my way of explaining my disease to someone who doesn't know, "Well, I have a disease called Eosinophilic Esophagitis. This disease limits the type of food I can eat. Currently, I'm on a _____ diet (elemental, elimination, Paleo), but hopefully I'll be able to add foods back in to my diet in the future." Now, after I explain, I have found that there are two types of people: the "satisfied-no-questions" people, and the "ah, that's interesting, I want to hear more" people. The "satisfied-no-questions" people will be content with your summary and won't inquire further, either because they're already too confused or they don't care and don't want to hear anymore. The "ah, that's interesting, I want to hear more" people are genuinely curious and really do want to hear more.

Word to the Wise: One thing I think is really important is asking your child how they want you to address Eosinophilic Esophagitis to other people. I told my parents that I would prefer them to explain it in such and such way. When I was younger, I was always worried that my parents were going to exaggerate or talk about an aspect of the disease that I didn't want to be talked about. So, I went up to them one day and talked to them about how I wanted them telling other people. It made me feel secure and confident. Just something to think about.

THANKSGIVING IN JANUARY

A lot of people ask me if my family eats what I eat, and I actually think the question is funny. I struggle with both sides almost every day. On one hand, why would my chicken loving, pizza eating family trade their Nestle Toll House cookies for some rice brownies? Sometimes I think they're so selfish when my dad makes eggs in the morning, (a personal favorite of mine). But, on the other hand, why would I be so selfish as to make them suffer through what I go through? Why would I be so selfish as to wish that they had to eat what I had to eat? I watch my mom try so hard, she's famous for her desserts. Her chocolate chip brownies, gooey butter cake, and pound cake are known around our friends and family. And every time she makes a dessert for my family, she always makes me something sweet too. Whether that's rice krispies, rice brownies, or tapioca cake, she always makes me something. And I know how hard it is for her to make them. Sometimes they don't turn out like they should. In fact, I usually have to scrape the brownie out, because it's stuck so hard to the bottom. But I love the joy in my mom's eyes when she's cooked me something that I enjoy.

A Tip and a Trick: If your parents care enough to try and cook you food that you can eat, go easy on them. There will be good recipes and bad ones. Just realize that they're trying and appreciate that.

Word to the Wise: Try your best to cook foods that your child can eat. Try to cook a variety of foods that will make your child feel appreciated and included.

THE GOOD, THE BAD, AND THE UGLY

When I've told people about my allergies and what I go through, they sometimes feel the need to give me advice. Which is ironic because how can someone give advice on something that they've never been through? The title of this chapter fits perfectly because I get advice from tons of different people, which are good, bad, or ugly. Sometimes I get advice that I know I will never take, I just smile and say, "Wow! You have such a good perspective. Thanks so much!" When I'm really thinking, "Oh my goodness. You have no idea. Stop telling me to make lemonade out of lemons when I'm allergic to the freaking lemon." Other times I will get good advice that has helped me through the rough spots. That advice didn't come from Dear Abby, the guidance counselor, or a heart-moving song. It came from someone who listened to me cry, knew my heart, and never got tired of me complaining. It was, and still has been, my best friend, Rachel Sproles. But believe me, she didn't meet me in one hour and start handing out advice the next. I met her in 5th grade, and then we lost touch until 9th grade. She didn't start giving me advice until my 11th grade year. Some people may think that's because we weren't close, or because she didn't care. It's quite the opposite actually; she took that time to just listen.

Now, you may be thinking, "What kind of advice is ugly advice?" Well believe me- there's lots of it out there. Ugly advice is advice that people say behind your back that you hear, but they don't know you hear. I've heard people whisper that I complain about my food allergies too much and I bore them. Well, I'm sorry if my disease isn't as important as who broke up with whom at the party. My point is, you'll get advice from tons of different people whether you ask for it or not. Personally, I don't like too much advice. Sometimes, some good advice seems bad, all because of the timing. I remember confiding in one of my very good friends about the hard time I was having. His advice was telling me how good I had it, compared to what some others were going through. Now, I look back on it now and think it's pretty good advice; but at the time, it hurt me more than it helped. I have to remind myself to have patience with people. I get so frustrated when people give me advice that I don't ask for. But keep one thing in mind- no matter how much bad advice someone gives, they give it because they care. Now I'm not talking about the ugly advice, that advice should be thrown away immediately and never looked back on again. But the bad advice you should appreciate. Trust me, I don't use 50% of the advice others give me. But it does make me feel a little better, knowing that they care enough to *try* to help me.

A Tip and a Trick: When that good little piece of advice rolls around, treasure it. It doesn't come around often, but you'll be thankful and welcome it with open arms when it does. And even though it's hard to treasure the bad advice, take solace in the fact that the person cares enough to try.

Word to the Wise: Be patient when other parents try to give you advice when they couldn't even imagine being in your shoes. Just smile and say thank you. That's about all you can do.

PART 2
(THE NO-FOOD LIQUID ELEMENTAL DIET)

BANGIN LIKE BRITNEY

So, after trying the elimination diet and still having allergic reactions, my parents and I made the difficult decision to put me on the elemental diet. In layman's terms, an elemental diet is an all-liquid formula diet. You take away all food from your diet and only drink a certain type of formula that is nutritionally fit. Think of it like this: when you go on the elemental diet, you're basically resetting your system. You're cleaning it out of all the food your body can't tolerate. You drink formula, and only formula.

When I found out that I was about to go without food for three months, I was pretty nervous, but I kept a good face for my parents. They applaud me for always being so strong and keeping a positive attitude. Well, let's get one thing straight: you won't always have a positive attitude all the time. As soon as I got in my car to drive to school, I felt absolutely powerless. I felt like I was

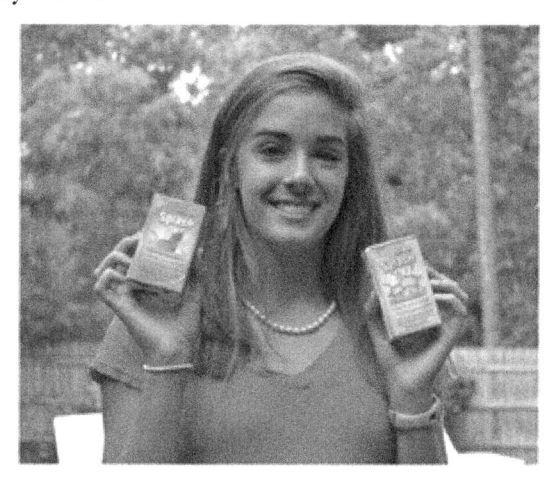

Above is a picture of me with the formula I drank, Neocate E028 Splash.

the weakest and smallest person in the world, and that everything and everyone was able to run over me. Food was taking over my life. I felt so weak. I knew from experience that I couldn't stay in this downfall too long, or else it would overcome me. I knew that I needed something to make me feel better. So, what did I do? I put on my Britney Spears CD. On that 15-minute drive to school, I sang and screamed that song until my throat was dry. It was my way of coping; my way of dealing with the news. Sometimes I scream to the music, sometimes I cry in my closet, sometimes I hug my dog, and sometimes I just take a nap. If I'm going to cry because I'm sad about the food I can't eat, then by the time I'm through, the whole pillow will be wet. If I'm going to be mad that no one knows what I'm going through, then I'm going to do so many pushups and get my anger out until my arms are worn out. I have no ritual that gets me into my peaceful world. It all depends on where I am, what the news is, and how it affects my life and my family.

A Tip and a Trick: Don't be afraid to show your emotions. I guarantee that if you have food allergies, and you have to start taking stuff out, or changing your lifestyle, it's going to be hard. You will feel powerless, weak, mad, upset, and betrayed. Each time you feel one of those, you have to figure out your personal antidote. And the antidote may change each time. Remember: you are not powerless.

Word to the Wise: Parents, realize that your kids need a way to deal with their allergies. You need to give them their space and let them cope their own way. And, not every time is our coping going to be the same.

FORMULA IMPORTANCE

*This piece is especially important if your tween/teen is struggling with drinking the formula.

Looking back at the beginning of April, I remember when I first started the liquid diet. I didn't know much about it, and I wasn't informed. From the doctors' information, I knew somewhat of how hard it would be, and the challenges I would face. But I didn't know everything. I wish I had had a book, a person, or an article preparing me for what I was about to dive head first into. That's really one of my main goals for writing this book. I want to help you make the best decision possible if you're thinking that you need to go on the elemental diet, or if you're a new beginner on the diet. Let me just say a few things that may not have crossed your mind before.

If you do not drink the correct amount of formula each day, bad things will happen to you. I am completely serious about this. When I first went on this diet, I thought the worst that could happen if I didn't drink all of my formula would be that I lost a few pounds. I didn't think it was that big of a deal. But I was completely wrong. Initially, when the dietician and the nurses tell you a specific amount of formula to drink, they aren't just picking a random number. They are basing it on four things: your weight, your height, your age, and your activity level. If you play sports on a regular basis, you are going to drink more formula because you need more nutrients.

When I went on this liquid diet, I thought the only thing that mattered was calories. I stupidly thought that I could have only 16 ounces of formula per day, which is 480 calories, and just drink a lot of slushies throughout the day to get in more calories. I didn't realize that I was missing something extremely important.

Nutrients. The stuff that keeps your bones strong, that keeps your heart pumping, and your brain thinking. When drinking less than 1/3 of the recommended daily amount of formula, bad things started happening. I started losing weight, my energy level dropped, I started getting very painful mouth ulcers, and I was horribly mean and aggravated. My body pretty much started to shut down. I didn't understand until I sat down with my uncle (who's a doctor) and he explained all of it to me. He told me how calories are only a piece of it; how, when I wasn't getting calcium, potassium, vitamins, or anything else, that I was hurting my body in unimaginable ways. I only wish that I had been told this sooner. I was stupid and immature. Don't make the same mistakes I did. If you're having a hard time drinking all of the formula, talk to your parents about it. Talk to the doctors about it. You're drinking the formula not to lose weight, or to look better, or anything like that, you're drinking it to survive.

And if you think drinking your formula each day is hard, wait until you start adding back on foods and are still required to drink the same amount of formula. As I'm typing this, that's exactly what I'm going through. I am still on the elemental diet, while trialing one food, corn. In the beginning I thought the addition of corn would lessen the amount of formula I had to drink a day…well I was wrong. I thought that when I started to add foods back on, I would be able to eat them as meals. My doctor up in Ohio quickly informed me that I could not just live off of corn, that I still had to keep up the same amount of formula, while only sampling corn. This is really hard, but what it teaches you is balance. To be able to balance the joy of a new food while still keeping the responsibility of drinking all your formula is something wonderful all on its own.

My point in writing this piece isn't to scare you. It is to tell you the importance of drinking your formula. I sadly did not realize the importance of it, and it hurt my body in the beginning.

A Tip and a Trick: Do not make the same mistake I did. Do not think that you can cut down on your formula intake. If you're old enough to be away from your parents, stay truthful and drink the formula when you're supposed to.

Word to the Wise: When your child is on the formula, sit down with them and explain why the formula is important. Explain why vitamins helps your body, what minerals are, etc. It may help your child understand it more, and why it is so crucial to drink the correct amount of formula.

A MONSTER IN DISGUISE

What's big, gets under your skin, and will never go away? That's right. Insurance companies. The biggest battle is the disease itself. The second biggest battle would be the insurance companies. They're big, bad bullies who will take every cent of your lunch money if you let them. The hospital fought and bartered with them. My parents are trying to get our insurance company to cover the liquid formula, but the insurance company is saying that it's not "serious enough." When my parents told me that, tears of anger started rolling down my cheeks. Why were they denying me? What had I done to make them do such an offensive crime? Not only was I taking on the burden of having no food in my life, but also now my parents had to take on the burden of paying for no food in my life.

My parents tell me not to worry about those companies that it's not my concern and all I have to do is focus on pushing through whatever diet I'm on. And while the food/formula is expensive, I hate that the insurance won't cover it. My family has already been burdened so much by my allergies; insurance not covering my medical health is just the icing on the wheat and egg free cake.

A Tip and a Trick: I know how frustrating the insurance companies can be. It's even more frustrating when they make life more difficult for your parents. But you really shouldn't worry about it. This is one problem that you can't solve or do anything about. So just let it go and leave it for your parents.

Word to the Wise: It seems like talking to your insurance company is fighting an uphill battle everyday. Try looking into advocacy groups in your state for Eosinophilic Esophagitis. Currently, there are 16 states that are forced to cover the liquid formula. I would suggest looking into those groups and seeing if your state is on that list.

BE YOUR OWN ROLE MODEL

I was sitting in the car, on my way back from Tennessee. My dad was driving and we started talking about my food situation. I felt so alone at that moment; feeling like no one knew how I felt. I knew my dad was trying to help; he was truly trying to reach out to me. That didn't matter at the time though. I just felt like I had such a heavy burden on my shoulders, and I was going to have to carry it for the next three months by myself. And, let's face it; there isn't a lot of encouragement someone can give you when you're going through a bad rough time. "That sucks," and "Oh I feel so bad for you," can only help a person so much. My dad was trying to reach out and help me, but it just really wasn't doing me any good. And then he said something, something that has stuck with me since then. He told me that I'm a role model for so many other people, and so many other people look up to me because of what I'm going through. I can honestly say I've never looked at it like that before. He told me that people admired how strong I was. Those few words completely changed my attitude. It now occurred to me, that not only was I doing this for myself, but also I was doing this for other people. Other people thought I was the strongest person they knew. And I couldn't let them down. The thought of being a role model to others rejuvenated me so much.

A Tip and a Trick: So, my small words of wisdom: Remember that people admire you for what you're going through. Know that you're a role model for others. Hopefully that will encourage you as much as it's encouraged me.

Word to the Wise: Tell your children how others look up to them for their strength and courage. It may inspire them and give them an opportunity to look at things in a new light.

ONE DAY DOWN

So as I'm typing this, it is my 3rd day on the elemental (liquid) diet. All seems well right now, and I emphasize the right now part. I catch myself having thoughts such as, "This isn't too bad, I could do this forever." But then I remember that this is only my 3rd day. I remember that this is going to go on for a few agonizing months. My knees then start to get weak, and I get tears in my eyes. Not because I'm scared, but because I realize how long this process is going to be.

Probably the weirdest thing I've had to do is re-train my mind. I catch myself looking forward to lunch because I can make myself something yummy. But then I remember that my yummy lunch comes in an 8-ounce juice box.

I realize just how consumed my mind was in food. I also realize just how obsessed I was with food. Anyways, I just think the most important thing in this whole experience is your mind. You have to have the right mindset in order to get through this.

In a way, I believe that if you're a teenager having to go through this, you have the benefit of understanding. Think about it. Most of the people that go on this liquid diet are babies and toddlers. For many, they don't understand why they have to go on this and take away all of their favorite foods, so they just refuse to drink it. This requires them to have a feeding tube. But, because we are teenagers, we know why we have to do this. Having the right mindset could save us from having to go on a feeding tube. Or, maybe if you're on the elimination diet, having the right mindset could save you from going on the elemental diet. Wherever you are on your journey, I thoroughly believe that having positive thoughts will get you far.

A Tip and a Trick: Take it one day at a time. It seems so much easier if I tell myself that all I have to do is get through today. It's so much better if at the end of every day, I pat myself on the back and say good job. Do not, I repeat, do not measure how many days you have left. Because when you're in the experience, days and months can seem like a lifetime.

Also, don't go into the kitchen when you don't have to. All that is going to do is make you wish you could eat something when you know you can't. Avoid going into restaurants at all costs. I made that mistake yesterday, and believe me, my stomach was growling louder than a sea monster.

Word to the Wise: If your child is going through this, please try to avoid cooking extremely smelly foods. Lasagna, for instance, would not be a wise food choice to cook when your kid is in the house. When my mom made that, all I wanted to do was leave. I got upset, angry, and hurt. When you're cooking dinner, try to remember that we can smell all that delicious food, but yet can't have even one spoonful of it.

A LITTLE SUGAR GOES A LONG WAY

Throughout this whole process, you have to keep some type of positivity in your life. Whether you've just been diagnosed with food allergies, you just had an allergic reaction and you're reading this in the hospital, or you have just been allowed to add foods back into your diet, you are not alone. I know how hard it is when I say to have a positive outlook through all of this. The whole idea of taking away food really has no positive angles. But, there are silver linings. What's a silver lining you might ask? A silver lining is that one thing that shimmers when you're surrounded by darkness. And, I truly believe with my heart that that is the thing that gets you through the darkest parts of any of the diets. A couple of days into my liquid diet, things were starting to get really hard. But then my doctors told me I could have Smarties and Dum Dums because it was basically just sugar and food dye. Believe me, I was about to jump right out of my pants. So, I had found my silver lining in a little plastic wrapper. I don't know how you'll find your silver lining, but I guarantee there is one out there.

A Tip and a Trick: Try to find your silver lining. Look for an opportunity presented to you in this time of darkness. I know how hard it is to be consumed by pain and weakness. But I also know that if you can find something to still smile about, you'll get through it a lot easier.

Word to the Wise: Talk to your child's doctor and see if they feel comfortable with allowing your child to have Smarties and/or Dum Dums. Most doctors are O.K. with it because it is artificial flavoring and sugar.

THE PARENTALS

Besides you, the people who must struggle through this process, who also hurt when you hurt, are your parents. Parents see all the 'behind-the-scenes." I know it's hard on them to watch me go through this, and they seem so weak sometimes. A lot of the time I feel like, in a way, I have to take care of my parents. I feel like I have to put on a charade in front of them, telling them I'm fine when all I really want to do is crawl into their lap and cry. Starting about 2 years ago, I knew I had to become stronger if I was going to get through all of this. Somewhere in the process, I also began to block out my parent's comfort.

Later on in life, I would find that my parents did not need comforting; they were strong as it is.

A Tip and a Trick: I know that what I wrote above says that I felt like I wanted to protect my parents. My advice? Don't always feel like you have to take care of your parents. Don't make my mistake. Trust me, they're stronger than you think. They have their own personal way of dealing with this, and you just have to let them work it out their own. Also, please be sure to go hug your mom, dad, grandma, uncle, whoever it is that takes care of you. They take a lot of time and effort and put it in to making you feel better. Don't be unappreciative. Thank them and let them know how grateful you are that they care enough to fight this nasty disease with you. I know that I need to thank my parents more often.

Word to the Wise: Parents, if your child acts like they don't want your comfort, chances are they probably do. They are just either too proud or too shy to admit it. I know it's hard, but be strong for your kids. Or pretty soon they're going to start feeling like they have to worry about you too.

THE SIBLINGS

Your siblings. Or whoever else is living with you. I have one brother who is 2 ½ years younger than me. We don't really have the closest relationship in the world, but we know that we love and care for each other. Whenever I've been on a diet, Matthew (that's my brother's name), has always been nice to me about it, but kind of kept his distance. I'm in no way saying that's bad. I mean, what else is he supposed to do? He's always been as supportive as he can.

When I went on this elemental diet, something changed in Matthew. He was still the same quiet little brother, but something had definitely changed. He was a lot more involved with my diet. He's the one who's told my parents to leave the room when they were eating something. He's been the one who has kept my juice boxes in stock. My point in saying this is to tell you that this diet changes people. It not only changes yourself, but it changes the way others think of you. It changes others' point of view. This diet has changed the way my brother thinks. It's changed our relationship, definitely for the better.

A Tip and a Trick: While you should be thankful for your parents, you should also be thankful for your siblings. They worry about you too. Your siblings are the only ones you've got, so treasure them.

Word to the Wise: If one of your other children wants to help with your child that has EoE, let them. Matthew wanted to help my mom in the process of cooking my food and cheered me on when I drank my formula. Let your other children be involved in the process, and it will create an inseparable bond.

SMELLS ALWAYS HAVE THE SAME EFFECT

When on an elimination diet or an elemental diet, you're restricted from certain types or all types of food. When on any type of diet, common sense would be to not be around the food you couldn't have because it's only going to tempt you to eat it and then it's going to be twice as hard. When I've been on elimination diets, I would always go to a place that I know could cater to my order and would have something that I could eat available on the menu. I knew that if I went to someplace like Chick-Fil-A (which has almost nothing safe for met to eat), I wouldn't have a good time because I couldn't eat anything on the menu. Now that I'm on the elemental diet, I try to avoid going out to restaurants at all costs because I don't like to be around any sort of food.

One question that I get asked a lot is, "If you're around food long enough, does it get easier? Does your craving for food eventually just kind of wear off?" The answer to that question is yes and no. Yes, in a way it does get easier. The longer you're on a diet, the more you remember that you're on it. Sometimes I'll still choose to sit at lunch with friends, and I don't even think about wanting a bite of that sandwich because I've been reminded for so long that it's not even an option. But on the other hand, it doesn't get easier. Just because I can handle sitting at lunch once in a while does not mean that I can handle walking into a buffet dinner room.

I'm on the track and field team at my school, and the day of regions meet, the head coach wanted to sign everyone out of school early and take us to this huge buffet restaurant in town and treat us to a free meal. Of course everyone was excited about this, not only about getting a free buffet meal, but also about getting to leave school early. When I heard, I immediately thought that I wasn't going to go. I knew I couldn't eat anything there, so I just made up my mind not to go. But as I started talking to some friends, they encouraged me to go. They just said I could sit there and talk with them. First off, this is a lot easier for them to say than for me to actually do. I don't think they realized this. I was pretty doubtful at first, but they convinced me to go.

As soon as I walked into the place, I knew I had made a bad mistake: steak, macaroni and cheese, chicken, pizza, bread, fries, brownies, ice cream, and chocolate cakes filled the air. The whole team walked back to our reserved spot. After everyone's drink had been ordered, people got up and went to fill their plates. I could only watch in agony. One by one, they came back with wings and pasta, steak and okra, pizza and fries, and ice cream sundaes. I watched everything. It was absolutely horrible. At that exact time, I remembered why I didn't like sitting at the lunch table, why I never hung out in the kitchen anymore, and why I left the room if someone brought in a food that I could see or smell. Sure, in a way my friends were right; I did talk with them (or more like I talked to them while they were stuffing their stomachs).

My mistake had been small but crucial. I simply thought that I could handle it and it wouldn't bother me too much. Boy, was I wrong. The whole time I was there, I just wanted to cry. It wasn't that I was mad at anybody in particular or anything, it's just that I was mad at the situation. I was mad that I had to have such an un-fun disease. I was mad that I allowed myself to come. I put myself into a situation that I immediately regretted.

A Tip and a Trick: If you're on a very restricted diet or an elemental diet, don't think you can just sit there with food all around you. I truly thought I could and it wouldn't be a big deal, but I was completely wrong. All it does is make you upset and uncomfortable.

Word to the Wise: If your family insists on eating out, order takeout so your child doesn't have to be surrounded by the smells. Eat it away from your child so they don't have to even see it. When I was on elemental, my parents ate in the closet to try and keep the smell as contained as possible.

THE STRONGEST SICK ONE

I was sitting in my 5th period Creative Writing class the other day, and the class was having an open discussion about my food allergies. They asked me questions, and my answers spurred more questions. It was a pretty good discussion, my teacher also contributed with stories of her own. She was telling us a story about a friend of hers who had some type of disease that I can't remember the name of. The disease was very hard on her friend and friend's family; having to watch their loved one go through something so horrific. My creative writing teacher made one interesting comment that really stood out to me. She said that the man (who had the disease) gave his family strength by his positive attitude. I thought this was so interesting. You would think that because he had the illness, his family would help him. But no; he had the illness, and yet he helped his family.

    I was thinking about this, and I still do all the time, and I've decided that that's how I want to be with my Eosinophilic Esophagitis. I want my positive attitude to be able to give hope to others. I know that it's hard on my mom and dad to watch me go through this. I want to be able to help them.

    One night on Facebook, I was talking to a friend, and I asked him what he thought about my food allergies. I wanted to know if he thought that I talked about them too much, or if I explained them in an awkward way, or if he thought it was scary. His response was just like the story above. He said he liked how I could joke about my allergies and talk about them light-heartedly. He admired how strong I seemed on the outside, even if I didn't feel like that on the inside.

    My thought is that if you keep a strong, positive attitude, your life will become easier. Listen, I said *easier*, not *easy*. People will admire your take on all of this. And even if you aren't light-hearted on the inside about this disease or allergies, try to be on the outside. It will encourage others so much.

A Tip and a Trick AND Word to the Wise: If you're looking for a way to change the outlook on your/your child's food allergies/disease, try being strong for others. In becoming strong for others, you may actually end up becoming stronger for yourself.

HAPPY MOTHER'S DAY

It's a few days before Mother's Day and call me a procrastinator, but I still had not gotten my mom anything. So after school I grabbed my wallet and headed for Target. I knew there was a specific watch she had been looking at, so I bought it and moved to another store, Tuesday Morning. My mom had seen some really cool cooking stuff, so I went in to check it out. Well, there was a ton of cooking stuff, so much that I just couldn't choose. A lot of it just blended in. Spatulas looked like whisks and knifes started to morph into spoons. I started scouring the aisles, looking for something that stood out, something that my mom would love. Finally, I saw it. There, the last one, in the very back, was a bottle of olive oil with peppers in it. I knew she would love this. As soon as I picked it up, memories came flooding back. One quick, easy snack that my mom loved to fix and eat with us was buying a loaf of French bread from the grocery store, then taking olive oil and putting it in a dish. She would then put some salt and pepper into the dish and mix it with the olive oil. Then, all she did was dip the bread into the olive oil and enjoy. This was, and still is, one of her favorite dishes of all time. So as soon as I saw that olive oil mix, I knew it was the jackpot. This would be perfect for the next time she fixes this snack!

As I was on the way home, a pure wave of emotion hit me. All I wanted was some of that bread dipped in olive oil. Just one bite; that's all I wanted. Suddenly I could just taste the saltiness of the olive oil hitting my tongue, the bread melting in my mouth. I hated that I couldn't have the privilege of what I was giving to my mom. Next thing you know, I was crying; I was so mad at the world. I was so upset, and I just hated it.

I felt like I only wanted just a little bit of food; anything. I felt so out of control. Like food was controlling my emotions. I hated it. I hated myself. I felt horrible. As I'm typing this, I still feel horrible, just not as much. I hate how food could bring such anger out of me. I'm embarrassed and ashamed. I feel so weak for letting food have this type of emotion over me.

Anyways, I cleared myself up before pulling into the driveway and walked in the door like nothing was wrong.

A Tip and a Trick: Always keep something with you to quickly eat. Whether that's a pack of Smarty's, an extra juice box, or a granola bar, keep something with you. I think if I had something in the car, it would have made me feel better. Another thing to keep in mind: times like this will happen. When you just feel completely out of control, mad, and upset. It's okay.

Word to the Wise: You may be wondering why I didn't really talk to my parents about my "true feelings." Maybe this is just me, or maybe it's like a lot of other teenagers, but I like to be strong. To show others that I am strong, and that includes my parents. Sometimes I don't like to tell others that I cry, or cry in public, because I want to be strong. I don't think this is bad. I know a lot of people that cry in private. I also don't like my parents to worry about me. They already do enough with my food allergies; I don't want them to worry even more. I'm not saying that this is how it should be parents, but I am saying that this is probably how your child thinks.

AHH, FRESH AIR

I know that throughout a lot of Part 2, I've complained about being on an elemental diet. I've told you how it's no fun, it's expensive, and it makes you feel frustrated. You might be turning the page, dreading reading another section because you're so tired of hearing negative side affects of this diet. Well, don't dread anymore! This section shows the positive side of this diet.

When someone has to go on this elemental diet, it's because something is wrong with them. Their stomach, throat, or intestine is messed up. Usually, this puts people in a lot of pain and they go to their doctor. Whether that pain is constant reflux, too many allergic reactions, choking, or whatever it is, it can get extremely painful. So the doctor checks you out, and long story short, diagnoses you with an Eosinophilic Disorder. For some people, they could care less and go about their normal day because they didn't have any pain in the first place. But for most people, it's somewhat of a relief, because they now have something they can blame for all of their pain. People with this type of pain usually want to get rid of it. With Eosinophilic Disorders, you can do one of three things. You can go on an elimination diet, an elemental diet, or steroids. People know that any of the three choices are hard, but the pain can become too much, so they'll do anything to get better.

When my family and I made the decision to go on the elemental diet, we didn't just do it because we thought it was worth a shot and if it didn't work, oh well. We did it because of how much pain I was in. I couldn't get through one day without there being some type of choking, reaction, or reflux. I was tired of going to the nurses and then being in bed for the rest of the day. (Keep reading, I promise I'm getting to the positive part).

Even though this elemental diet has been hard, it's also been one of the best things that has ever happened to me. I can't tell you how proud and happy I feel that I have not had one allergic reaction since I've been on this diet. No more knife-stabbing pain, no more throats closing, no more choking. I don't wake up in the morning wondering what foods are going to try to hurt me today. I may be a little hungry, but I'm pain free and worry free! To someone who is in immense pain by the foods that they eat, this is a wonderful thing.

When you go on the elemental diet, you have many different formulas to choose from. My favorite is the EO28 Splash, which comes in a little juice box. Other options include big canisters of formula, which you can blend with ice. About two weeks into this diet, my dad asked me what it was like to drink the formula that came in the juice boxes (EO28 Splash). I thought about it for a little bit, and told him that when I took that first sip, it was like I was getting a breath of fresh air. Like my body was so happy to have that formula again that it just sent a shock through my system jumping up and down for the arrival of the amazing liquid. My taste buds may have hated it, but my body was so relieved that it was still getting nutrients without the harsh side affects.

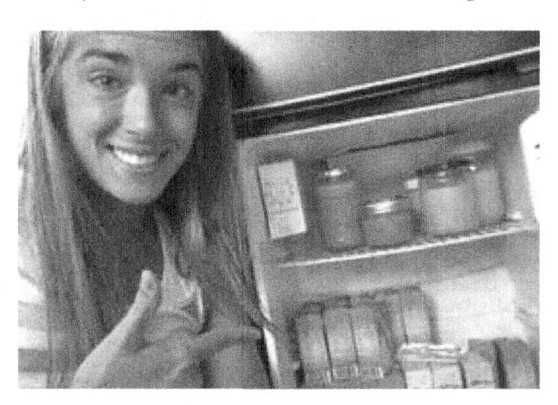

Above is a picture of me with my persona; mini-fridge and all of my formula!

1*A Tip and a Trick: If you're on the elemental diet, try to view the formula as a breath of air. It's giving you energy, nutrients, and essential vitamins for your body. It is helping your body. Think of it as replenishing and nourishing.*

Word to the Wise: Depending on your child and the kind of formula he/she has, try to spin it in a positive way. Blend it with ice to have a smoothie or put it in a Starbucks cup to have a "frappe." My formula was in a juice box; so it may me feel just a little better.

LOUD AND PROUD

Another thing that I think is important through this whole ordeal is feeling proud of yourself. I remember I was sitting in the car on the way to a doctor's appointment, and I was just feeling really down about myself. I told myself I was such a sissy for being upset that I couldn't have a certain food when people were fighting cancer every day. I was beating myself up, not giving myself any credit. People tell me daily about how strong I am and how they could never do what I do. I guess I never really listened to them. Partially because I had heard it a thousand times and partially because I'm more used to it so it didn't seem as big of a deal to me. Recently, I had a mini-revelation. I realized that I am strong, I am a survivor, and I should feel proud of myself. I have accomplished so much. I'm not trying to brag, but what I'm saying is that you should give yourself credit where it's deserved. Beating yourself up all the time and telling yourself how weak you are is only hurting you, not making you stronger. I know that I thought that if I told myself that people went through so much worse that would give me the strength to drink the nasty liquid. But no, that's not what gave me the strength. Telling myself that I'm strong and that I can do this, that's what got me through. I've often thought of this disease as a selfish, one-on-one type of thing. I know my parents and friends try to help and comfort me, but I know that in the end, it's what I tell myself that will make a difference. Someone can tell me all day how proud they are of me, but if I don't believe that and tell that to myself, then it's not going to make a difference.

A Tip and a Trick: Be proud of yourself and what you've been through. Don't down yourself by saying that you're a wimp or you should be tougher. Give yourself a break. Don't throw a pity party, but don't be too tough on yourself either. It's okay to recognize that you're a survivor, and you'll pull through.

Word to the Wise: I know when I was younger, I would make comments to my parents like, "I'm sorry I'm complaining too much," and "I'll just be quiet now, I'm a wimp." If your child makes comments like that, something deeper is probably going on. Tell them that they are strong, and that they should be proud of themselves because not many people could be as strong as they are, waking up and not eating foods. Show them how proud you are of them. It'll make a difference.

JUST A LITTLE BITTER

I was on the couch one night talking to my mom, and the conversation came up about my food allergies and my thoughts about others and food. I guess I had never really thought about it until I said it aloud to her, but I told her that I don't pity people who want some type of food but don't get it. I also told her how much I dislike picky eaters; my mom must have recognized the power in my voice because she said something that really took me by surprise. She told me to not be bitter, and to not be callous. At that moment, I realized that I was. I was, and still am, bitter about not eating. It's not an outward trait that I show to everyone, but it's definitely there in the back of my head.

What I don't think is fine is if you show your callousness or bitterness to others. Now I understand every once in a while, you snap at someone who complains about a food that they don't like. It happens to the best of us when we're either really tired, really hungry, or both. But if you constantly persecute people because of their eating habits, their eating choices, or their eating complaints, then people won't want to be around you (even if you're right).

I know that being on this liquid diet has changed my perspective in so many ways. Because I can't eat food anymore, when I go over to people's houses, and they complain of there "being nothing to eat," I get so angry because they have no idea what they're saying. In fact, I even get mad writing this.

One thing I've learned about being on this diet is that I've become so much healthier. I've learned truly what my body needs, like vitamins and minerals. I've made promises to myself, that if I'm ever privileged with the opportunity again to eat whatever I want, that I will only eat what's good for me. Most people have the privilege of eating foods every day, all day. And then, partly consciously, partly unconsciously, they choose to use their privilege and hurt themselves in the process.

A Tip and a Trick: I personally think it's okay to get annoyed when your friends are picky eaters. "At least they get to eat" is the first thought that runs through my head. I think it's natural to get annoyed, just don't let that annoyance consume you. Don't let it make you bitter.

Word to the Wise: Do what my mom did. Tell your child to not be bitter. I didn't even realize it until someone else pointed it out to me. Try to keep your child as well rounded as possible, and to not just focus on their problems.

THANKSGIVING IN MAY

So, you probably read "Thanksgiving in January," which is in Part 1. Now since I'm on the elemental diet, I'm writing a, "Thanksgiving in May." This piece is another way for me to give thanks. Now since I can't eat any food, it's very hard for me to be around food at all. My family has realized this, and now they don't eat around me ever. You may say that that's pretty hard for them, and you're right; it's extremely hard for them. But they do it because they love me. If they're eating and I walk in the room, they'll either leave the room and go outside or go to a different room. They plan their big meals and cookouts for when they know that I'll be at a friend's house or away. I'm so thankful for this.

A Tip and a Trick: If you know your family is planning a cookout or something big, plan to go hang out at a friends or go to the mall. You don't want to be around the grilled chicken or the smoked vegetables.

Word to the Wise: think about them when you're eating. Now I don't mean feel guilty, because I know I don't want my own parents to feel guilty for eating, but think about eating in front of them. Try not to do it. It means a lot when my family puts in the effort to not eat around me; it shows me that they care.

BECOME A BUSY BEE

I think one crucial thing that has helped me get through the absence of food is always doing something. I have learned that when the average person is not doing something, or they are doing something but they're bored, they often turn to food. And why not? Eating food makes most people happy, it entertains most people, and it takes up a whole lot of time. When I first started this elemental diet, I had a lot of free time on my hands. This free time was suddenly created because drinking a juice box took about 20 seconds, not 20 minutes. I started to find myself just sitting at the lunch table, on the couch, or on my bed; my mind consumed with the thought of food. My mistake here was doing nothing. Because I was doing nothing, my mind wandered off to food.

Have you ever had a really busy Saturday? You woke up, went somewhere, ran some errands or did some chores, picked up some milk, met your friends at the movies, and then babysat the kids next door. Sometimes you just kind of forget about food until you stop and think, "Wait, I haven't had lunch today." You were so busy that you just didn't really notice that you were hungry or that you didn't have food. These are the best kind of days for me. When I forget about food.

When I got on the elemental diet, I stopped going to lunch because I couldn't stand being around so much food. So, what did I do? I filled up that extra 25 minutes. I have started going to other teacher's classes and offering to grade papers. I've started sitting outside and listening to people play their guitar. I've started coming to the library to finish some of my homework.

With all this free time, I've become so much more productive throughout my day. At home when I'm bored, I'll clean my bathroom or bedroom. I'll start a project a few days early, or I'll clean the car. Whatever it is, I know that I'm getting something done and being productive.

I would have to say that this has actually benefitted me in a lot of ways. I'm helping teachers out, I'm meeting new people, and my grades are becoming better because of my additional focus in my classes.

A Tip and a Trick: Start becoming busy. And when I mean busy, I mean don't let yourself have any free time whatsoever, until you go to sleep. Sometimes in classes, you get bored with your teacher's lectures and you start to think about lunch. Well, for someone who doesn't really get lunch, this will only make you hungrier. Pay more attention in classes. Put all of your focus into every single word the teacher is saying. Make your notes as detailed as possible. If you put your whole mind into the class, then I guarantee you'll stop thinking about food. I also recommend not sitting at the lunch table. When I was on the 6-food elimination diet, I could do it and was fine with it. But when I was put on the elemental diet, I could no longer watch people enjoy their peanut butter-and-jelly sandwiches with their Diet Coke and cupcake. I tried it at first, but it wasn't fun and I didn't need to put myself through it. Once again, this has required the right kind of thinking. A big portion of this journey is acquiring the right mindset. It's taken me a good year to accomplish this, but I promise that when you do, everything will get a lot easier.

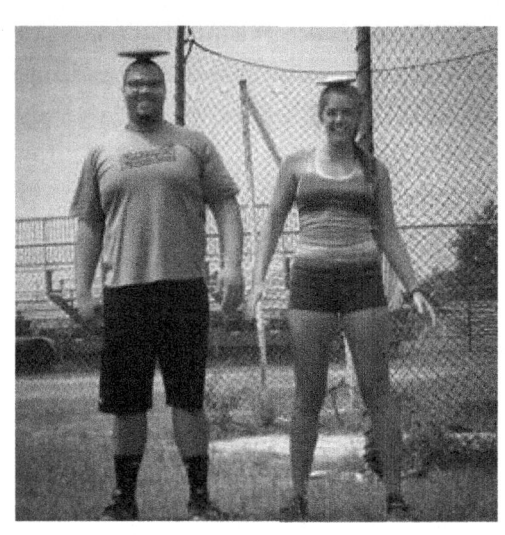

To stay busy, James and I would throw discus and occasionally take a goofy picture!

Word to the Wise: Keep your child busy. Don't let them mope on the couch. There's a difference between low energy and moping. If you can keep your kids entertained, keep their focus on something else, then I promise that you'll see a difference in their spirit.

JUST COUNT BACKWARDS FROM 100

I have about six surgeries under my belt, and since I'm 16 years old, that means I have somewhat good experience. I'm not really nervous anymore when I'm about to go under, because I know exactly what's going to happen. (My purpose in writing you this is to give you an idea of what's going to take place and how to make the best of it).

Now, the first thing you need to know about surgery, is that there are two types. There are inpatient and outpatient. Inpatient surgery would be when you have to spend the night at the hospital. An outpatient surgery, commonly referred to as an outpatient procedure, is where you don't have to spend the night at the hospital. Endoscopes are usually outpatient and are relatively short. Depending on the experience of your doctor and depending on the specific type of procedure done, you can estimate how long yours will take. My scopes in Georgia took about 15 minutes, and I was out for a total of about an hour. My scopes in Ohio have been done in less than 10 minutes, and I was still out for about an hour.

About a week before the surgery, you should know your schedule. Every hospital is a little different, but the standard is to get a schedule of when your scope will be, and when your pre-operation (pre-op) visit will be. Pre-op is just when you come in about an hour to an hour and a half before the scope and meet your doctors, change into your gown, and get set up. I've always liked pre-op just because it's a good time for me to relax and focus.

On the day of your scope, remember not to eat or drink anything. Once again, every hospital is different and has different rules about not eating or drinking before; the general rules of thumb is no solid food 8 hours before and no clear liquids 4 hours before. Don't forget to check with your doctor to be sure. I remember for one of my scopes, I drank some Sprite about 4 hours before my surgery and I had to wait an extra 30 or 40 minutes because the doctors didn't want to risk anything. It's always better to ask than to chance it.

Also remember to bring something to do. I like to bring my iPod to listen to. Hospitals get pretty crazy and sometimes the wait is longer than expected. Listening to music helps me relax and not become nervous. I said in the beginning that I don't get nervous a lot anymore, but that's only partially true. I still get a little nervous, but nearly as much as I used to. My brother loves to talk about everything and make small talk and constantly chatter, while I just want to ignore the world and concentrate on my music.

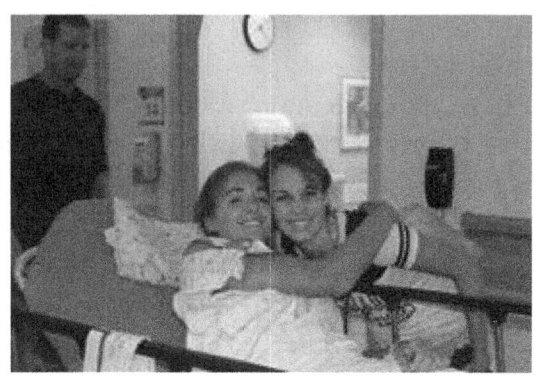

Above is a picture of my best friend, Rachel, and me as I was about to go in for a scope. Dad is photo-bombing the background.

See if your hospital has a little toy section. Most children hospitals do, and I know it's always fun to pick out something. Granted, most of the toys are for little kids and aren't really that good, but sometimes in the back I've found a Bath and Body Works lotion or a cute teddy bear. That's another thing, being 16 years old, I'm technically still a child, therefore on the pediatric side. Sometimes I feel weird; I feel so large when I'm surrounded by a bunch of toddlers. But I'm actually very glad I'm still in the children's section. The children's side seems to be a lot more happy and carefree.

A Tip and a Trick: I definitely recommend wearing some comfy clothes. It doesn't really matter since you'll have to put on a gown anyways, but when you have to get re-dressed afterwards, it's a lot harder to button up your jeans than to slip on some sweatpants. Also, I like listening to powerful music before my scopes. I like feeling like I am a little bit in control, and listening to strong, powerful music makes me feel good. That may not be your technique, but find something that you like and bring it with you to your scope.

Word to the Wise: Parents, when I get nervous, I get really quiet. I just kind of stop talking and zone out into my music. At first, my parents wanted to talk with me and socialize with me before the scope, and would get frustrated when I just really didn't want to talk. Realize that each of your children have a different way of dealing with anxiety, and respect it. Also, make sure to bring any and all important forms and documentation. Write down all of your questions before, so you can go in and ask the doctor all of them and not forget one.

JOURNEY (NOT THE SONG, SILLY)

Everyday is a journey; a journey with new lessons to give. I have new opportunities thrown at me, and meet all sorts of people. I meet bad people who judge me before they know me, but I also meet good people who make a difference in my life.

Yes, it's sad that I have to say this, but people will judge you and make jokes about what you go through. I've had people taste my formula and say, "This tastes fine! I don't see the big deal about it!" *Not a big deal?* I would say to myself. *Then you try living on it.* I've had people make fun of the juice boxes I drink and call me a little kid.

A Tip and a Trick: The only advice I can give you is to either walk away or stand up to them. If you walk away, don't keep everything bottled up inside. Go talk to your best friend about it. Tell them how it hurt you beyond belief and whatever else you're feeling. If you're going to stand up, make it straight and to the point. Tell them that it's not cool what they're saying and they have no idea what you've been through. Let them know that until they have EoE, they can't comment on your life. No matter what you do, just know that you're the only one who knows how you feel. Don't let someone tell you that you should stop being a baby or just get over it. They have no idea what they're talking about, and they aren't worth listening to.

Word to the Wise: While it's sad, the harsh reality is that as your child gets older, they will probably get teased for drinking formula, or for having a feeding tube, or for eating weird foods. Encourage your child to recognize that they're different, and to own it. My EoE and my food allergies have made me different, special, and unique. Talk to them, and tell them how they should be proud of who they are, and what they've accomplished.

TO GO ELEMENTAL OR NOT? THAT IS THE QUESTION.

This piece goes out to the teenagers and families who are questioning whether or not to go on the elemental diet. I was once in your shoes. I had tried a lot of diets, including the 8-food elimination diet, and it just wasn't working. The elemental diet was right there, but it seemed so big and mysterious. I wish that when I had to make the decision, I could've talked to someone who had been there, done that to help me think it through. Besides the doctors, my parents and I were flying blind as to what to choose. We really had no choice left but the elemental diet. For many families, the elemental diet is usually the last resort because not only can it be expensive, but also it's hard to stop eating. Plain and simple. It's hard to watch your child not eat. It's hard for the child to be around food and not eat. I remember when I was on the fence about wanting to do it or not. I remember telling my parents that I wanted to do it because I was tired of having allergic reactions and I wanted to feel safe when I ate food. But I also remember telling them that I was afraid of how hard the elemental diet was going to be. I knew that the formula didn't taste the best, and a lot of kids had to get a feeding tube, but I really didn't know how hard it was going to truly be.

Part of the reason why I wanted to go on the elemental diet was to lose weight. This wasn't a really big deciding factor, but it was definitely something that was in the back of my mind. I was a 16-year-old girl who was 5'10 and weighed about 150 lbs. I was in no means overweight. I didn't think I was really fat or anything, I just wanted to lose a few pounds to look good for summer. Hear me loud and clear on this: Do not do this elemental diet to simply lose weight. I do not advise this or recommend this in anyway. Being on the elemental diet, I've lost a few pounds, and nothing has really changed. I thought that if I dropped a few pounds, then my life would be perfect. People would like me more, school would be more fun, you know, just everything would be better. Well, I was wrong. Nothing really changed except for the fact that my jeans were a little looser. And the fact is that if you start losing a lot of weight on this diet, the doctors are only going to make you drink more because the point of this diet isn't to lose weight, it's to heal your esophagus.

A Tip and a Trick: If you're having a tough time making that final decision, try asking yourself these questions. "Is this the last option? Have we tried all other elimination diets?" "No matter the amount, am I going to be able to force myself to drink it?" "Am I going to be able to handle this emotionally?" For some, they don't care and they just want to get better. For others, they may rather be in pain than take away their food. For me personally, I was tired of going to the hospital, not being able to swallow foods, and living in general fear of what I ate.

Word to the Wise: If you and your family are considering putting your child on the elemental diet, you not only need to consider how hard it'll be for your child, but you need to look at the financial aspect of it. There are only a handful of states that require insurance companies to pay for formula. The only way that all states require insurance to pay for formula is if your child has a feeding tube. So, for example, I live in South Carolina. The state does not require that insurance pay for the formula if your child takes it orally, but does require insurance to pay for it if your child has a feeding tube. Neither my parents nor I wanted me to have a feeding tube, so my parents took on the burden of paying out of pocket for my formula, which is extremely expensive.

PART 3
(THE PART ADDING FOOD BACK ON ONE AT A TIME)

INTRODUCTION

For any of you who have been on or are thinking of going on the elemental diet, then you know, or will know, that the best part of an elemental diet is what comes next- adding foods back on! After three months of no food at all, it can be pretty exciting to add a food back into your diet. There are so many foods out there that it can be dizzying. But not to fear, you have me here! Some doctors suggest referring back to your food allergy test and picking a food based on what tested negative...I on the other hand don't really agree with allergy testing, and therefore pick foods based on their nutritional value, doctor's recommendation, and overall likeability of the food. For me personally, I added on corn as my first food, then beef, and then sweet potatoes and blueberries. In this section, I talk about the feelings of elation when you get to add back on your first food and how adding back on foods is more difficult than you might think.

THIS OR THAT, DOC?

The day before the big day. The big day is the day of the first scope after being on the elemental diet for three months. Now, for a girl who has had multiple scopes and surgeries, having another scope isn't really that nerve-racking. It's not something that really bothers me; I know exactly what's going to happen and I'm pretty comfortable with the whole thing. But, the day before this scope, I was as nervous as a turkey before Thanksgiving Day. (Pretty good analogy isn't it?)

This scope was so much more important than the others. My previous scopes had been more of a diagnosis and a confirmation of Eosinophilic Esophagitis more than anything else. Since being on the elemental diet for three months, this scope would determine if I still had eosinphils in my throat. If they were gone, then I could add back one food and so the long process of trial and elimination would start. If the eosinophils were still there, then the doctors would know that it wasn't being caused by food, but by my body itself, and would give me steroids. There were so many "what-ifs" for this scope and so many questions that couldn't be answered until after the scope.

A couple of hours later, I'm in the recovery room, waking up to the distant sound of my heartbeat.

I slowly start waking up in the recovery room, coming to the realization that it's over, that the results are here, and I should know the results in a couple of minutes.

My favorite nurse is talking to my parents. I can hear her sounding quite joyful and that gives me a lot of hope.

Once I'm fully awake and talking, I ask them what Dr. Putnam said. *Drumroll please!* He said that there were no eosinophils to be found! Which means that it was food causing the eosinophils, so I can add back on one food at a time and find out which exact foods cause the eosinophils. When I heard this, I was ecstatic. For the first time in my life, my esophagus looked the way a normal esophagus should. I knew that I didn't want to be on steroids for the rest of my life. And now, I could start eating corn! Yes, corn was what I asked to be my first food back.

If you're on an elimination or elemental diet, and you are preparing for your scope that allows you to add on another food, research some food beforehand to see what you would personally like to add back. I chose corn because corn comes in so many varieties; corn, creamed corn, popcorn, grits, corn chips, corn tortillas, homemade corn bread (it would have to be homemade depending on if you couldn't have items like wheat and eggs) and corn muffins, etc. The list goes on and on.

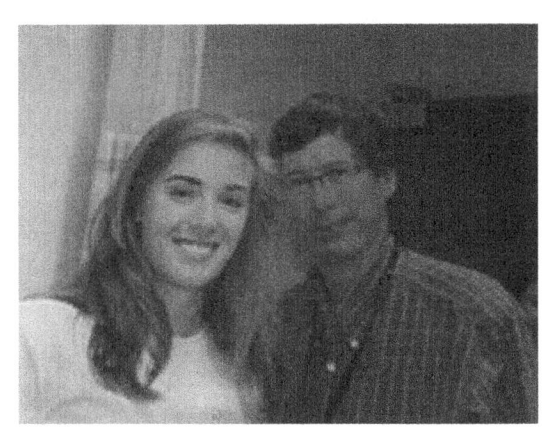

Dr. Putnam and I before a scope!

A Tip and a Trick: If you're about to try and add on another food to your diet, get excited! With any food, there are endless possibilities out there. I tried to do a meat, a starch, and a fruit to keep it balanced.

Word to the Wise: When helping and determining what food your child is going to trial and try to add back into their diet, keep in mind the versatility of the food. I chose corn originally because of its versatility. Pumpkin seeds, on the other hand, would be harder to trial just because of their lack of versatility.

DEFINITION OF WEAKNESS

Everyone has their weak moments. And you better believe that you'll have them whether you're on the elemental diet, the elimination diet or any diet for that matter. The longer you're on the diet, the easier it gets. But let me make one thing clear. "It gets *easier*" not, "It gets *easy*." Those are two words that sound pretty similar but have two totally different meanings.

In the beginning of each of my diets, the first few weeks were pretty hard. My body had to learn to readjust and to adapt. Personally, I believe one of the most remarkable qualities of the human body is adaptation. After a couple of weeks, the body slowly starts to adapt and learn whatever the new normal is; you start to accept it.

Make no mistake though, being on an elemental or an elimination diet doesn't "get easier" overnight. In fact, it's such a slow change, that you probably won't recognize it until you're months into it.

For me, at first, each and everyday is hard. (I warned you in the beginning of this book that I would not be all fluffy and frilly. I would give you the facts and a true inside look at my life). In the beginning, each day is a constant reminder that you either cannot eat a whole list of foods, or that you cannot eat any food at all. And after a few weeks of constant dread and wishing you could just sleep through it all, these reminders start to fade away. Sometimes it'll just be at lunch, when you don't even think about wanting food- just because you're not really hungry and don't want to eat. Other times, you'll be with your friends for a few hours, and not once will the thought of food cross your mind. And then, slowly but surely, food will leave your thinking process. In the morning, you won't think about grabbing a granola bar or cereal, it just kind of skips your brain. At lunch, it'll start to become a habit to not go to the lunch table, but instead outside or to the office or the gym. You'll still have hard times, my experience being most often at night when I'm tired, but they hard times won't be as often.

As I'm typing this, I'm in my 4th month of the elemental diet, with one food back, corn. I still hit rough spots, like when my family goes out to dinner, or when I couldn't have cake on my birthday, or when I'm simply just tired and fed-up with everything. But the rough spots become so distant that living with this becomes a lot more manageable.

When I'm going through a tough time, my best friend tells me something that really encourages me. "Being strong doesn't mean you're never weak. Being strong means getting through the weak parts and coming out stronger." This may sound cliché, but in a time of sadness and madness, it really does help.

A Tip and a Trick: Take the advice of Dory from Finding Nemo: just keep swimming. I understand the hard days. But understand me when I say that they will pass. One day, you will get semi-used to this lifestyle. One day, it'll be your new normal.

Word to the Wise: Keep your eyes on the future- don't wallow in today's misery, but know that one day it will get better. Yes, the elemental diet is hard. Yes, some days are worse than others. But it will get easier, I promise. Just stick through it and be strong.

THE DEVIL IS EVERYWHERE

*Some people may not like this chapter. Some people may not think that people cheat on diets. If you are one of those people, then this may be especially helpful to you. Kids will try to sneak food; 6 years old or 16 years old, they will try. So read this, or get your child to read this. I promise it's worth it.

When you're six years old, your parents are always one step ahead of you. They usually pick out your clothes, make your meals, take you to play dates, and pretty much manage your life. If you're on this elemental diet and you're six years old, your parents are probably in charge of everything. They give you all the formula and make sure you drink all of it. They don't drop you off at the mall, or watch you drive off to your friend's house. No, they are with you almost all of the time. But if you're reading this, and you're like me, a teenager who is on this elemental diet, chances are you have a lot more freedom. If you're too young to drive, you probably are still allowed to go hang out at a friend's house. If you're old enough to drive and have a car, then you definitely have more freedom. My point in saying this is to make you aware of how much freedom you have, and to talk to you about the dangers of cheating. When on any type of diet, there is always temptation. Everywhere. And believe me, when you're on a very strict diet of little food or no food, temptation can come in the form of anything starting with apple pies and ending with zucchini.

Now you may think, "What's the point of having an accountability partner if I've already done the deed?" (And by deed I mean eating a food you're not supposed to have). Well, this type of partner isn't the kind that you confess to. This type of partner is one you go to *before* you cheat. If you're in a situation where you know you're about to eat something that could either hurt you or mess up a scope, then you need someone you can call when you're in need. I have just recently gotten an accountability partner who I can call anytime I need them. My close friends would tell me how it's not worth it, they would keep my mind off of food, and they keep me from making a big, potentially harmful mistake.

The second thing you need to do is stay away from temptation as much as possible. Now does that mean staying locked in your room and never coming out? You may think that, but no, I'm talking about staying away from restaurants or parties with a lot of food. (And while I agree to not torture yourself with all this food, it's not all I'm talking about. I believe the biggest temptation is when you are by yourself). When you're at a restaurant or a big party, sure there's food, but there's also a ton of people around who know you can't eat food. They are your "temporary" accountability partners. But, when you're by yourself, that's when the big temptation is. No one is around. No one will know. One bite could make a difference. All it takes is one bite.

The third and final thing that I believe is really important is to always keep something to eat or drink with you, in case you're ever super hungry. When you're extremely hungry, you become irrational. You grab a handful of raisins and swallow them so quickly before you realize that you're allergic to raisins, or that you're not supposed to eat raisins. So, if you on an elimination diet, always keep an emergency food with you. If you're on an elemental diet, always keep a little bit of formula or some Smarties with you. (I say Smarties because my doctor in Cincinnati allowed me to have Smarties while on the elemental diet because it consists of artificial flavoring and sugar. But please, check with your doctor beforehand to make sure it's okay).

A Tip and a Trick: Take it from me personally, when you get on this diet, or if you're just starting out, you need to do three things: One, get an accountability partner; Two: stay as far away from temptation as possible, and Three: always keep something with you to eat or drink.

Word to the Wise: I know this is upsetting, but the chances of your child cheating, or trying to cheat, are extremely high. I know how frustrating that is because not only are you spending money on the formula/expensive rare foods, but you're spending time trying to heal your child. My parents would get so upset when I told them I ate something I wasn't supposed to. And believe me, I felt horrible. Not only horrible physically, because the food I would eat would make my stomach churn, but I would feel horribly guilty and shameful. I knew I had disappointed my parents and let them down. So, while it's frustrating, try to also have mercy. Talk to them about why you don't want them to cheat, explain how it's costly and how it hurts their body. Also, try to keep temptation away from them. Don't leave a fresh batch of cookies on the counter. If your child cheats, talk to them. Don't get angry, but talk to them. Figure out ways that you can help them to not cheat.

CONCLUSION

Adding food in and taking food is a life-long process for children and adults with EoE, or any food-related disease for that matter. You'll have safe foods and danger foods. Your safe foods are the foods that don't give you any problems, and/or have been tested and have found no eosinophils. Your danger foods are the foods that you know give you trouble, and/or have been trialed and found to produce eosinophils in your throat. Foods that you know give you trouble but enjoy once in a while anyways. Sometimes, in order to give your body a break, you'll take away all of your "iffy" foods and just stick with your safe foods. A new danger food may be discovered and immediately you stay away from it. It's one of those things that you'll have to do. You constantly need to be listening to your body, seeing how foods make you feel, and adjusting. But really, that's what life is about; adjusting and readjusting.

PART 4
(ANOTHER DIAGNOSIS)

WAIT...WHAT?

In the introduction, I said that this book was written over a span of four years…when I was 14, I was diagnosed with EoE. I started writing when I was 16, and when I was 19, I was diagnosed with something called Ehlers-Danlos Syndrome. In this section, I will go into detail about Ehlers-Danlos Syndrome; what it is, how it is diagnosed, how it's connected to EoE, and what symptoms I had. I am including this part in the book, because I don't think it pertains to just me. An association between the two has been forming a strong bond over the years, and I think it's worth mentioning.

SO, WHAT IS IT?

First off, Ehlers-Danlos Syndrome is not a disease. It is, simply put, a collection of symptoms that affect a body. (That is the definition for any syndrome). For this specific syndrome, it affects the connective tissue of the body. Connective tissue includes your blood, cartilage, ligaments, and tendons.

There are six main types of EDS (Ehlers-Danlos Syndrome). The most common type is Hypermobility, which is Type 3. Since this is the most common type, and the type I was diagnosed with, it's the only one I'm going to go into some detail about. The other five types of EDS can affect your heart, intestines, and blood. If you're concerned that you or your child has one of these types, I encourage you to visit www.ednf.org to learn more information.

Type 3, Hypermobility, is a type of Ehlers Danlos that affects your cartilage. It can make you very flexible, but not in a good way. In layman's terms, your thumb cartilage may be able to bend very easily, but then may not be able to "snap back" causing damage to the cartilage because it's too stretched out. In the next few pages, I'll go into some more detail about my symptoms and how I was diagnosed.

AM I BREAKING?

"Am I breaking?" This is the question I was starting to ask myself all of the time. Around the age of 18, a lot of changes happened. I started my freshmen year at the University of South Carolina (Go Cocks!). I also started my freshmen year on the University's track team. Since I had loved throwing the discus in high school, I decided that it was time to take that passion on into college.

I loved throwing on the track team. My new college coach was a highly respectable man who taught me just as much about life as he did track. I enjoyed the atmosphere as much as I enjoyed my teammates, and I just loved the experience. After a few months of training though, something started to feel wrong. I was always in excessive pain, never feeling 100%. Throwing felt harder than it had ever been, something always felt pulled or torn or sprained, and I just didn't feel up to speed. I hesitated talking to my coach or to the trainers because I didn't want to complain. I thought the pain was in my head and I pushed forward. I could feel myself getting weaker and weaker by the day but I had no clue why.

I finally mentioned it to the track trainer, who told me to go get some blood work done. I did, but the blood work came by fine. I was told to eat and sleep more and I would be fine.

Long story short, after months and months of ignoring my pain and pushing through, I got tired of it. Throwing was

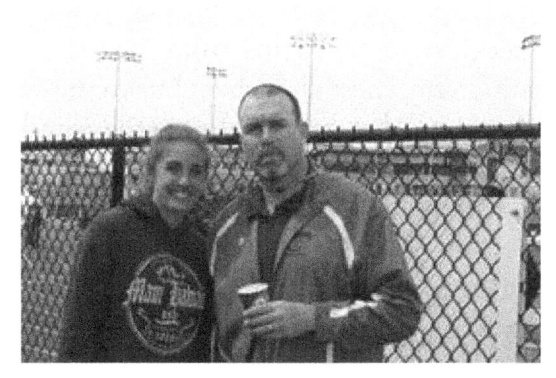

A picture of my college coach, Mike Sergent, and I right before I competed!

no longer a relief to me but a chore. I started to resist in the weight room because it was so painful. The summer after my freshmen year of college, I resigned from the team. I told my coach that I respected him too much to represent him in something that I wasn't passionate about. It was a rough decision, but I knew it was the right one.

It's truly ironic the way things happen in life. I had always thought that the pain was in my head, and I just had to push through it. I quit the track team in May when the season ended; however, my body was still hurting after May. I wasn't working out extensively or throwing…so why was I still in pain? And before I go any further-let me clarify what "pain" I am talking about. My wrists were in pain, my toes were in pain, and my chest was in pain. It hurt to cut steak with a knife. It hurt to sneeze. It hurt to run. It hurt to walk. It hurt to hiccup. It hurt to push open a door with the palms of my hands. So, as you can imagine, I was highly confused and frustrated. Believe me, if you had an intense pain in your chest every time you sneezed or hiccupped, you would be frustrated too.

So, because my parents are wonderful people, we started going to doctors again. I saw a rheumatologist and had MRI's done on my chest and wrists. The results were interesting to say the least. In my chest, I had a piece of inflamed cartilage in between my rib and my sternum. The doctors said that it was probably inflamed from my excessive weight lifting from the months before. This explained the pain in my chest and why it hurt to move it. I also had very small, but very many, tears in all the cartilage in both of my wrists. The doctors also said that this was because of my throwing the hammer and the discus for so many years with such intensity. This explained why I no longer opened doors with my hands or cut meat. They said that if I stopped lifting, the cartilage should heal itself. The aggressor (lifting and throwing) was no longer present, so therefore the cartilage would not have any other reason to be aggravated. The doctors said that it should take my body about six weeks to heal.

Six weeks came and went, and I was still in the same position that I was in in May. My mom called the rheumatologist, who said three interesting words, "Ehlers-Danlos Syndrome." My mom then called the infamous Cincinnati Children's Hospital, and asked them about it and if they had ever heard of it.

This next part is my favorite- Dr. Putnam (the man who I will always think of as a miracle doctor), called my parents personally and talked to them for about an hour on the phone. For any of you who have experience with doctors and hospitals, it's hard to get in touch with a nurse let alone speak with the doctor for more than 10 minutes. So when he made a personal house call to talk to my parents specifically, that meant a lot. Basically, he told them that there was a lot of new research being done linking EDS and EoE. He said that the two were highly correlated with one another, and if a child had one diagnosis, there was a very distinct possibility that he/she had the other. He then suggested that I come up to Cincinnati immediately and find out if I had EDS. My parents' agreed, and next thing I know I'm in the backseat of the car making the 10-hour drive to Ohio.

When we finally arrived in the cloudy town, I met with a whole team of doctors. They measured my flexibility, hyperextension, and pain levels. I met with pain management doctors, psychologists, and many more. At the end of the week, it was determined that I had type 3 (hypermobility) EDS.

When I was diagnosed with EoE, I was relieved. I finally had an answer to my problem. I felt the same way when I was diagnosed with Ehlers-Danlos Syndrome. Yes, I was scared. Yes, I was confused. But I was mostly relieved. To have an answer for all of the pain can truly be a surprising weight off your shoulders.

A Tip and a Trick: Listen to your body; you know it better than anyone else. If something is hurting, speak up! Don't doubt yourself like I did, but instead trust your body and yourself.

Word to the Wise: If your child tells you something is wrong, listen to him or her! Chances are, they probably aren't faking, and they can probably feel something, they just don't know how to explain it.

SO NOW WHAT?

So I came back home, and asked myself the question, "now what?" I now have two different "body struggles" (I refuse to call myself a diseased person). Since you can't really fix or cure EDS, physical therapy was recommended to help strengthen the muscles around the joints. Let me say- physical therapy definitely helped. I was more than a little leery at first. I mean come on; I went from lifting 200 pounds. and now you want me to squeeze a ball fifteen times? Please. Those were my exact thoughts the first few times I went. But after a while, surprise surprise, I started feeling better. My wrists were healing up, as well as my chest. It no longer hurt to sneeze or cut a steak. Because of my EoE, I couldn't take traditional oral medications for the pain. Instead, I was given medicine that is administered through electricity and ultrasound. It sounds kind of scary, but it helped me a lot, and to this day, I still go back when I have flare-ups.

A Tip and a Trick: For any teens reading this specific part: no matter how stupid you think a treatment is, please just do it. As a former athlete, I know it seems redundant, but just do it. For me.

Word to the Wise: In the beginning, I was really resistant to physical therapy. I truly did not want to do it, and did not see the benefit of it. This is where my parents had to be tough, and tell me that I was going to do it, or I was going to sit in pain for the rest of my life. I encourage you that once in a while, as hard as it seems, to be tough with your child. I know that I needed that "toughness" to get me to see the benefits of my physical therapy.

PART 5
(THE TECHNICAL PART)

DEATHLY HALLOWS OF INSURANCE

As I have been writing this book, I've been waiting to finish the last part: Insurance. I haven't wanted to leave anything out, and the monster of insurance is definitely not something to ignore. For the readers who are trying to become more informed about the elemental diet, formula is expensive. Formula is even more expensive when you choose the type that is flavored. You may say, "Expensive? As in blueberry juice expensive?" No. I'm talking liquid gold expensive. I'm meaning like every eight-ounce juice box filled with white, thick formula costs $4.25. In the beginning, when I was on completely liquid, I had to drink 64 ounces a day (8 juice boxes). 8 juice boxes times $4.25 equals $34.00 dollars a day. So, when I say it's expensive, trust me, I'm not joking. Naturally, you would assume that health insurance would pay for this kind of stuff.

But they don't. Only a handful of states have made it law requiring insurance to pay for formula. South Carolina (where I live) is, of course, not one of those states. Meaning that my family's health insurance does not want to pay for my juice boxes and formula. Seeing as how it could get quite expensive over the years, my dad has protested and hired a lawyer to fight our insurance company. Well, I got the news today that the lawyers can no longer fight the case, because there is no case. The insurance company "denies" me. When my parents told me this, many many things went through my head, 99% of them that I cannot write about. I was so genuinely angry. I still am. How dare they say, "I'm not sick enough to be covered"? I can't eat food for crying out loud!

A Tip and a Trick: Please do not let the insurance companies upset you. As much as you feel like it's your concern, it's not. It's your parents' job to worry about insurance and formula costs, not yours. Let them be parents and let them do their job.

Word to the Wise: See if your state is under the policy that mandates for your insurance to pay for the formula. Not all states are, but it's worth looking into.

HOW TO HANDLE THE HOLIDAYS (OR ANY SPECIAL EVENT)

When it comes that time of year, it's hard to celebrate with your family while having food problems. I briefly wrote about this earlier in the book. I talked about food alternatives and ways to avoid food. I want to talk about one more way to handle the holidays (Halloween, Easter, Thanksgiving, Christmas, Hanukah, Kwanza, the whole sha-bang). Every year for our family reunion, my entire extended family goes down to the beach. Our favorite family tradition is to go to the local crab shack and stuff ourselves silly full of fresh crab. Unfortunately for me, I love crab. It was unfortunate because at the time, I was on my elemental diet. There was no alternative to crab, and there was no way I was going to sit at the table and watch everyone eat my share of crab. So, my mom did what she does best. She took me away for some "me" time. We went walking on the beach, shopped at the local stores, and watched the sunset. These were all activities that I loved, and they got my mind off of food. It was a simple way to make me feel like I wasn't missing out on anything.

A Tip and a Trick: Ask a parent if you can have an alternative to sitting at the big family dinner table while everyone eats. Or, if it's crucial that a parent must be there, then maybe do something for yourself; paint your nails, read a magazine, anything.

Word to the Wise: You and your child can do anything- whatever he/she likes. Take them to a skateboarding park and let them show you his new moves. Take them to the new movie. Anything will take the focus away from food, while also giving you and your child some quality time.

STEREOTYPES: THERAPY

I put this piece in the Technical part because I feel like it could be for anyone in any stage of where they are with EoE. I also named it Stereotypes because I feel like there are a lot of stereotypes that come with the word therapy.

Right when you hear that word, I know 10 different thoughts pop up in your mind. My child is fine. They aren't messed up. They don't need it. My personal favorite- I'm here for them if they need to talk. Personally, I think if your child is struggling, or if you're struggling, you should give therapy a try.

When I was going through my elemental diet, I was really angry. I didn't feel like I could talk to my parents or my friends about it. Eventually, I told my parents I wanted to talk to someone. I was nervous to tell them at first. I didn't want them to be upset or shocked that I couldn't talk to them. I just wanted an unbiased opinion from a stranger. My parents agreed that I needed to see a therapist to get some professional advice and help me sort through my feelings....I spoke with a family psychiatrist. My mom and I sat through the first half of the first session together so she (the psychiatrist) could have an understanding about our family

While I didn't stick with it for the long run, the few times I went were extremely beneficial. The sessions didn't magically make me happy. They didn't cure me. But they gave me new perspectives on how to think. They did make me think about things in a new light.

A Tip and a Trick: Overall, don't knock it until you try it. Therapy gave me new ways to think about things. It doesn't make you weird, or a failure, or anything. In reality, it'll probably make you a more enlightened person.

Word to the Wise: If your child comes to you and says that they would like to speak to someone, don't take it personally. It's not that they don't like talking to you, but sometimes it's nice to get someone else's opinion, or to talk without fear of judgment. Be supportive that they even want to talk and express their feelings in the first place.

THE SWEET SEVEN

My creative writing teacher suggested that I have a section including some of my favorite recipes when I was on the elimination diet. I thought this was a pretty good idea, excect my mom didn't know any really good recipes right off the bat. We had to search the Internet and ask around to find out some good recipes. So, instead of giving you some favorite recipes of mine, I'm going to give you some favorite brands of mine.

When trying new foods on your elimination diet, keep this in mind: you will taste some nasty food. Sometimes when companies try to make gluten-free cookies, they wind up tasting like cardboard-filled cookies. I have to give some credit to those companies because, hey, at least they tried!

This piece is also based on my personal preference. You may try some of these brands and think that I'm crazy for liking them.

I will try to save you from not trying too many bad foods to get to the couple good foods. And, you know, when on this elimination diet, you have to be somewhat brave. When my mom would cook new rice pasta, I had to be brave and hope for the best. Sometimes it was for the best, and sometimes…well let's just say the trashcan enjoyed it very much.

One more tip: when on any of my diets to try and help my EoE calm down, my family and I would go to the local health store and fresh food market and just go to town. We would get everything I needed for breakfast, lunch, and dinner. After buying everything, we would go back home and fill up my very own little cabinet. Day after day, I would try new things from my cabinet. Around the end of two weeks, my dad would go back to the health store and get me some more food. The problem? My dad would go back to the store to get me more food when my cabinet was still half full. My cabinet would still be half full because there was stuff in there that I tried, which had just been downright nasty. I just couldn't take it. But we had bought 3 boxes of it. The lesson of this mini-story? When buying foods, only get one box, just to see how you like it. Because if you don't like it, then you're going to have an excess of it which will go to waste.

Here are some of the brands that I've tried and have personally loved:

1. Any of the *Betty Crocker* brands for cookie mix, pancake mix, and brownie mix are really good. My mom has found that these are the easiest to bake.
2. *Ener-G*. (This is an egg substitute, so when you're making you gluten-free cake, and you can't use eggs either, you use this).
3. Most *Frito-Lay* chips are gluten-free
4. *Chebe* products. *Chebe* is bought online. They have many different products like sandwich buns, pizza crusts, bread sticks, etc. *Chebe* is pretty good; it just takes some time to learn how to cook it just right. *Chebe* is gluten, soy, rice, nut, wheat, and yeast free.
5. *Cherrybrook Kitchen* has really good cookie mixes, which are nut, egg, gluten, and dairy free.
6. *Galaxy Nutritional Foods* has really good dairy and soy free cheese. It's made from rice, and doesn't taste that different.
7. In this case, I have saved the best for last. I think the best chocolate chip cookie would be by the brand, *Home Free*. These cookies are already cooked, and come in individual packages. They are chocolate chip cookies that are gluten, egg, dairy, and nut free. These are really the best.

*Please keep in mind that these are just my opinions of some yummy foods. You may need to substitute more based on your specific dietary needs.

REMEMBER ME!

Here are a couple of key things to remember when you're on an elimination diet or an elemental diet. These lists of important things include things I think you should remember emotionally and technically.

When on an elimination diet, remember:

1. Explore all food options. There are tons of substitutes out there; they just might not be as highly advertised.
2. Don't listen to people who make fun of your food.
3. Look on Facebook for a page for food allergies. These pages usually supply good recipes that you can try.
4. If you cheat, you're not a failure. But, you do need to tell your parents or the doctor so they can set your scope date. Cheating and not telling anyone can delay treatment and give you false results.
5. It's okay to feel sorry for yourself once in a while.
6. Clear out a space, a drawer, a box, or a cabinet for your food.

When on an elemental diet, remember:

1. Drink lots of water. You'll be tempted not to drink water because you're already drinking liquid formula, but it's critical that you stay hydrated.
2. Talk to your doctors and find out if you're allowed to eat any type of hard candy (like Smarties or Dum-Dums).
3. Take everything one day at a time. Don't get caught up in the fact that you still have a long time to go before you can add a food back on. Get caught up in the fact that you've already accomplished so much already.

4. If your doctors allow you to have some type of hard candy like Smarties, *do not overload*. A high concentration of sugar in a short amount of time can make you get a super bad sore throat, super fast.
5. When on the elemental diet, I got colder quicker. In my opinion, it helps to bring a sweater along wherever you go.

A BRIEF STORY

One very important thing I've learned through this whole journey is that I meet people who I impact, and they impact me. If I didn't have this disease, then I wouldn't have the opportunities that I have today.

It all started when I filled out a scholarship application for a free trip to Washington, DC. In the end, I got the scholarship and was awarded by winning a free trip to Washington, DC for 6 days with 46 other students from South Carolina. We all went up and met up with 1,500 other students from 47 other states. Let me just say, the experience was amazing and I wouldn't trade it for anything in the world.

As the week went by, I made friends that I know will last me a lifetime. Of course, people saw me not eating and only drinking the formula. Naturally, they asked why and I think I explained it about 46 times. It took a little while, but by the end of the week, they understood why I couldn't have food, but why I could have blue raspberry slushies (it's because of the artificial flavor and sugar). They said that my story inspired them, and they would never forget me. Little did I know, that they would be the ones that I would never forget; the ones who inspired me.

I'm telling you, special things will happen to you if you accept your challenges.

On the second to last day of the trip, we were on our way back to the hotel, when the bus stopped. It was such a huge bus, and I was so tired from all the activities we had done that day that I simply didn't notice and really didn't care about stopping. I was about five seconds away from falling asleep sitting up. A few minutes after we had stopped, something went around my eyes. I didn't know what it was, but like I said earlier, I was so tired that I just either didn't notice it, or I just didn't care.

Next thing I know, something large and cold is thrust into my hands. The blindfold that had been wrapped around my eyes is removed and what do you know? I'm presented with an extra-large blue raspberry slushy. Seeing that slushy in my hand….it was more than just a slushy. I know it may sound odd, but the slushy represented just how much those people I had met four days earlier cared for me. They had made the effort to talk to the bus driver, find a gas station, stop, and buy me a slushy- one of the only things I could eat, and something that I had been craving since the beginning of the trip.

This is just one example of the cool things that can happen to you, if you just accept the facts of life. One important thing that I really want to stress in this book is that opportunities will be presented to you that you would never have had if you were not diagnosed with EoE. Now, I'm not saying that your life is so awesome because you have EoE. I know it's difficult. I'm right there with you. But what I am saying is that, if you let yourself, you will be blessed in so many ways.

Another blessing that I wouldn't have received if I didn't have EoE was when everyone went to the food court at the mall for dinner. I didn't (and still don't) like to sit with everyone while they ate, so I moved around, looking at the different kiosks set up. There was one necklace kiosk that I really liked. It probably had about 2,000 different necklaces and bracelets. I looked around for a few minutes, picking out funny ones, and unique ones, and serious ones. Soon I started talking to the man

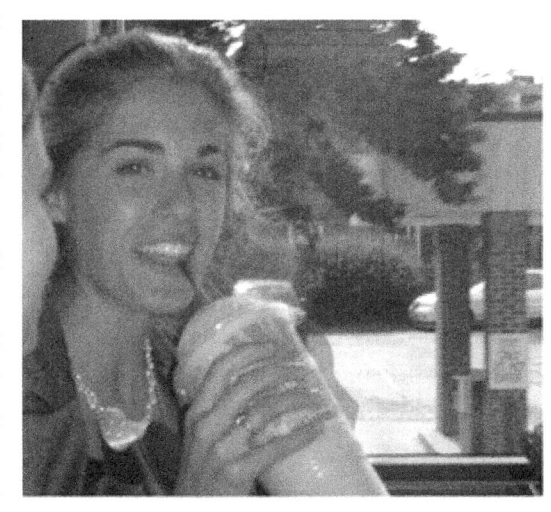

It's not the best quality, but it's the only photo that was taken with the blue slushy that my friends had gotten me. I was so overwhelmed with happiness!

working the kiosk, and he started showing me different styles and new shipments that they had just gotten in. There was one bracelet that really stood out to me. It was a silver charm bracelet, and all the charms were different food items. There was a hamburger, an ice cream cone, French fries, a soda, etc. I thought this was extremely ironic and quite funny and I decided that this was what I wanted. He asked me why I picked that one out, and so naturally I told him briefly about why I liked it so much and why I wasn't eating with my friends. I remember him just looking at me with bewilderment and astonishment. After asking some of the usual questions, he did something very unusual. He gave me that bracelet. I asked him if he was sure, and he said that he was the manager and he could do what he wanted. After that, I was the one who was bewildered and astounded. I couldn't believe it! It made me feel so special and happy. I think that God gives me these little gifts and opportunities as reminders that I do make an impact in others' lives and I need to stay strong. One way that I stay strong is through the support and encouragement of others. It was just too cool. And little did I know, that the best was still to come. Even writing at this exact moment, I know I have big things ahead of me. So do you. Just use your disadvantage to your advantage.

A few weeks after the Washington, DC trip, I got e-mail and a phone call from the company that had given me the scholarship to go to D.C. He explained in the e-mail that he was an editor for the national electric cooperative magazine, and he had heard about me on the Youth Tour. He said that he loved the story I had; about how I overcome my challenges and am still able to go on throughout my day. He said that he wanted to have an interview with me and run my story in the national magazine. Wait, hold up. National Magazine? Wow. This was huge! When he told me all of this, I was so excited. I was going to have the opportunity to share my story with over 33,000 people. These things just don't happen every day.

I wanted to share this story with you, so you know that good things do come out of bad things; that even after a thunderstorm, look out for the rainbow.

REFERENCES

Want more information? Check out these helpful websites.

1. American Partnership for Eosinophilic Disorders; www.apfed.org
2. Campaign Urging Research for Eosinophilic Disorders; www.curedfoundation.org
3. Food Allergy and Anaphylaxis Network; www.foodallergy.org
4. GERD; www.aboutgerd.org
5. MayoClinic and WebMd have also been great websites.
6. Cincinnati's Children's Hospital for Eosinophilic Disorders; www.cincinnatichildrens.org/svc/alpha/e/eosinophilic/fs/default.htm

THE...NO, I DONT WANT IT TO BE THE END

So, all good things come to an end, right? I mean, this book can't just go on forever. I don't really want to end it, because I'm sure I have thousands of more stories that are in the back of my mind somewhere.

Hopefully, my experiences gave you an inside look as to how hard having food allergies really is. Maybe you learned something new that you never knew before. Maybe I've given you some insight into what your child is going through. If you're someone who has bad food allergies, or an Eosinophilic disorder, keep this book handy. Write in the margins of it. Write down your feelings, what you're thinking. I truly believe that I'm going to be okay, just because I know that I'll be able to write everything down. Who knows, maybe there'll be a Volume 2 to this book.

My final words? Stay strong. As the saying goes, "The grass isn't always greener on the other side, it's green where you water it."

Made in the USA
Columbia, SC
03 January 2022